Atkins Diet Book for Beginners 2024

A Complete Guide to Healthy and Delicious Recipes with Easy-to-Follow
28-Day Meal Plan to Lose Weight + BONUS!

28-Day Meal Plan + Video Course!

Dr. Valerie Kennedy

Copyright © 2024 by Dr. Valerie Kennedy

Disclaimer!

The information provided in this [book/article/website/etc.] is for general informational purposes only. While every effort has been made to provide accurate and up-to-date information, Dr. Valerie Kennedy makes no representations or warranties of any kind, express or implied, about the completeness, accuracy, reliability, suitability, or availability of the information contained herein for any purpose. Any reliance you place on such information is therefore strictly at your own risk.

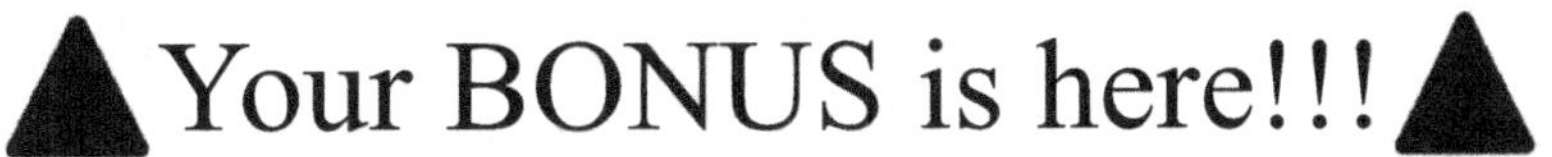Your BONUS is here!!!

28-Day Meal Plan

Induction (Days 1-7):

Breakfast:
- Keto Mini Chocolate Chip Muffins
- Keto Crustless Spinach Quiche

Lunch:
- Roast Beef, Red Bell Pepper and Provolone Lettuce Wraps
- Keto Garlic Ranch Dressing

Dinner:
- Maehing's Chicken Eggplant Casserole
- Keto Steaks with Green Onion and Caper Sauce

Snacks:
- Endulge Keto Chocolate Cups
- Atkins Chocolate Slushies

Ongoing Weight Loss (Days 8-14):

Breakfast:
- Keto French Toast Casserole
- Fennel, Carrot and Turkey Hash

Lunch:
- Keto Crab and Avocado Salad
- Keto Chili-Beef Kebabs

Dinner:
- Tofu Sautéed with Green Pepper, Scallions and Tamari
- Curried Fish and Red Peppers Over Broccoli

Snacks:
- Raspberry Parfait
- Atkins Chocolate Slushies

Pre-Maintenance (Days 15-21):

Breakfast:
- Keto Italian Frittata
- Keto Sweet and Salty Almonds

Lunch:
- Turkey Tacos
- Keto Summer Chicken Salad

Dinner:
- Keto Baked Tofu with Cajun Rub
- Wild Salmon Vera Cruz with Grilled Asparagus and Watercress

Snacks:
- Keto Mascarpone Parfait
- Atkins Chocolate Slushies

Lifetime Maintenance (Days 22-28):

Breakfast:
- Keto Crustless Broccoli Quiche
- Chocolate Pancakes

Lunch:
- Keto Beef Burger with Feta and Tomato
- Keto Spice-Rubbed Lamb Loins with Cucumber Salad

Dinner:
- Keto Chocolate Caramel Pretzel Cookie Bars
- Keto Chocolate Ganache Macarons

Snacks:
- Atkins Chocolate Slushies

- Endulge Keto Chocolate Cups

Here is one of the biggest bonuses I promised you…

A full video course on the **Atkins Diet**

To get access to it, kindly type in this link on your browser:
http://tinyurl.com/mpvp8zuk

OR

Scan the below QR code to gain access.

About The Author

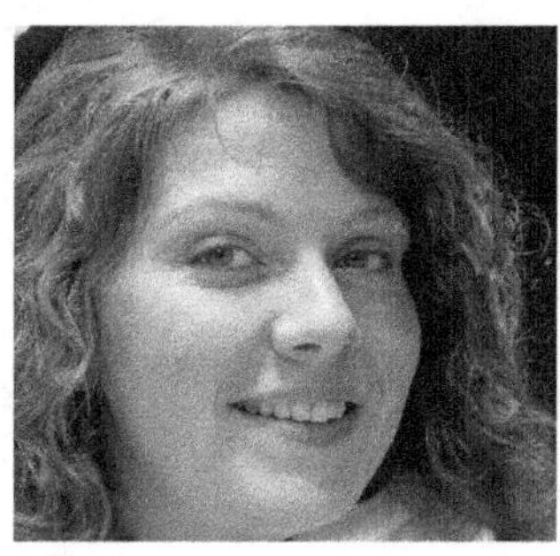 Renowned culinary expert and Culinary Institute of America alumna Dr. Valerie Kennedy is well recognized for her creative approach to food and in-depth knowledge of the many nutritional components that are included in every dish. For almost two decades, Dr. Kennedy has been a fixture in Michelin-starred restaurants' kitchens, showcasing his ability to blend traditional methods with contemporary, worldwide flare.

As an author, she celebrates the variety of cultures in her recipes while highlighting the link between our general health and what we eat. Dr. Kennedy's viewpoint on food is distinct since he considers cooking to be an artistic endeavor that feeds the body and the spirit, rather than merely a practical skill.

Connect with Dr. Valerie Kennedy:

Email: ***drvaleriekennedy@gmail.com***

Table Of Content

Introduction

Welcome to the Atkins Diet's world. We will go into great detail about the Atkins Diet in this extensive guide. It is a well-liked and successful weight reduction plan that has assisted many individuals in reaching their health objectives. This book is especially designed for beginners in 2024; we've included the most recent findings and trends in nutrition to provide you the most recent knowledge together with delectable, simple-to-follow recipes.

The low-carb, high-protein, moderate-fat Atkins diet was created by Dr. Robert C. Atkins and has been shown to aid in weight loss and general health improvement. There are four stages to the diet: the most restricted phase is phase one, and the next phases progressively allow you to reintroduce more carbs into your diet.

You will find a comprehensive guide to the Atkins Diet in this book, which includes:

1. *An outline of the advantages and guiding principles of the diet*
2. *An in-depth description of the four diet stages*
3. *An extensive inventory of items to consume and steer clear of*
4. *A 28-day food plan customized for you*
5. *Recipes that are tasty, nutritious, and simple to prepare*

You'll quickly achieve a healthy lifestyle and a smaller waist according to the recommendations and meal plans in this book. Now let's go on this thrilling adventure together!

The Atkins Diet is a low-carb, high-protein, moderate-fat diet that emphasizes cutting down on carbs while consuming more proteins and healthy fats. The idea behind the diet is that by cutting down on carbohydrates, your body will go into a state of metabolism known as ketosis, where it will start using fat for energy instead of carbs.

The diet consists of four phases:

Induction Phase: The induction phase of the diet, which is the most restricted, is meant to jump-start your weight reduction by allowing you to consume no more than 20 grams of carbohydrates daily. You will concentrate on eating veggies low in carbohydrates, healthy fats, and high-quality protein throughout this period.

Ongoing Weight Loss (OWL) Phase: Until you achieve your personal carb tolerance level—the amount of carbs you can eat without gaining weight—you will progressively increase your daily carbohydrate intake by 5 grams each week throughout the OWL phase.

Pre-Maintenance Phase: You'll begin the pre-maintenance phase after you're within 10 pounds of your target weight. During this phase, you'll keep adding 10 grams of carbohydrates to your diet each week until you achieve your target weight.

Maintenance Phase: You'll keep your target weight throughout the last stage of the diet by eating a body-friendly ratio of fats, proteins, and carbs.

Benefits of the Atkins Diet

There are several advantages to the Atkins Diet for those who want to become healthier and feel better all around. Among the diet's main advantages are the following:

Weight reduction: Many individuals lose a large amount of weight quickly on the Atkins Diet, which is a very successful weight reduction strategy.

Better Blood Sugar Control: The Atkins Diet, which lowers carbohydrate consumption, may help those with type 2 diabetes manage their blood sugar levels better.

Lower Risk of Heart Disease: Eating more healthy fats may help lower cholesterol and lower the risk of heart disease. This is why the Atkins Diet is recommended.

Enhanced Energy: A lot of individuals who follow the Atkins Diet report having more energy and having better mental clarity, which is probably because their bodies are now using fat instead of carbohydrates for fuel.

Decreased Cravings: The Atkins Diet may aid in reducing cravings for unhealthy foods by boosting the intake of healthy fats and proteins and regulating blood sugar levels.

Foods to Eat and Avoid on the Atkins Diet

It's crucial to concentrate on eating nutrient-dense, low-carb meals that will support your weight reduction efforts while adhering to the Atkins Diet. We'll give you a thorough rundown of what foods are allowed and prohibited on the Atkins Diet in this chapter.

Foods to Eat:

- Proteins: Make sure you eat enough of high-quality proteins, such organic eggs, wild-caught fish, free-range poultry, and grass-fed cattle.
- Healthy Fats: Include foods high in healthy fats in your diet, such as nuts, seeds, avocados, and coconut and olive oils.
- Low-Carb Vegetables: Vegetables low in carbohydrates, such as leafy greens, broccoli, cauliflower, cucumbers, and zucchini, should fill up your plate.
- Dairy: Select dairy items with added fat, such heavy cream, cheese, and butter.
- Fruits: You may indulge in low-carb fruits like melon and berries in moderation.

Foods to Avoid:

- Refined Carbohydrates: Steer clear of processed carbs like sugar, pasta, and white bread.
- High-Carb Fruits: Fruits heavy in carbohydrates, such pineapples, bananas, and grapes, should be avoided.
- Starchy Vegetables: Reduce the amount of starchy vegetables you eat, such peas, maize, and potatoes.
- Sugary Foods and Beverages: Steer clear of sugar-filled meals and drinks including fruit juice, soda, and candies.
- Processed Foods: Avoid processed foods like fast food, chips, and frozen meals.

<h1 style="text-align:center">Grocery Shopping for Atkins</h1>

The Low-Carb Dietary Atkins Grocery List

Stock up on the items you'll need to maintain a successful low-carb diet before you go on your Atkins weight reduction adventure. Having a stocked refrigerator with low-carb items will make it easy to prepare tasty and nutritious meals. Use this straightforward Atkins low-carb shopping list as a reference the next time you visit the grocery store! For Atkins 20®, Phase 1, the Atkins approved list of low-carb foods is another useful tool for selecting the appropriate meals and portion sizes.

Example of a Shopping List with Low Carbs

This is just a starting list for low-carb groceries.

Produce

- One of the main components of the Atkins Phase 1 diet is vegetables, which should provide 12 to 15 grams of net carbohydrates daily. When you reach Phase 2, you may start adding certain fruits.

Salad Bases

Add one or more of these leafy greens to your salad to start:

- Romaine lettuce
- Iceberg lettuce
- Arugula
- Spinach
- Endive

Snacks

In contrast to high-sugar chips or cookies, these snacks will support hydration, lightness, and refreshment:

- Celery
- Cucumber
- Peppers

Salad Toppers

Who declared salads to be uninteresting? Add some of these fresh ingredients to it:

- Mushrooms
- Avocados
- Artichokes
- Radicchio
- Radishes

Side Dishes

The ideal complement to any meal heavy in protein

- Broccoli
- Brussels sprouts

- Okra
- Snow peas
- Collard greens
- Eggplant
- Mashed cauliflower or cauliflower rice

Seasoning

Season any dish with these Atkins-approved spices to add flavor:

- Parsley
- Chives

Meat

The first phase of the Atkins diet allows for all meat. Here are some suggestions:

Meat

- Bacon
- Beef
- Ham
- Lamb
- Pork

Fowl

- Chicken
- Cornish hen
- Duck
- Turkey

Seafood

In Phase I of Atkins, all fish and shellfish are permitted. Here are some suggestions:

Fish

- Salmon
- Tuna
- Trout
- Cod
- Halibut

Shellfish

- Clams
- Crabmeat
- Mussels
- Oysters
- Shrimp

Dairy

The following dairy products are authorized to provide a creamy touch to any meal:

- Sour cream
- Mayonnaise

Cheese

Taste these mouthwatering cheeses as a snack, over meat, or on a salad! Each is authorized for Atkins Phase 1.

- Blue
- Cheddar
- Goat cheese

- Cream cheese
- Feta
- American cheese
- Gouda
- Mozzarella
- Parmesan
- Swiss

Refrigerator Staples

Always have these on hand for a delectable finishing touch:

- Eggs
- Salad dressings
- Lemon juice
- Lime juice

Pantry Staples

To save time while preparing meals, stock up on these essential culinary supplies:

- Chicken or vegetable broth or bouillon cube
- Splenda
- Vegetable oil
- Olive oil
- Herbs and spices
- Avocado oil
- Coconut oil
- Low carb hot sauce

Beverages

Although water is necessary, the following drinks are approved by Atkins Phase 1 for when you want to switch things up:

- Flavored zero-calorie seltzer water
- Diet soda
- Club soda
- Coffee
- Tea
- Club soda

Chapter 1: The Science Behind the Atkins Diet

Your body uses fat and carbohydrates as fuel. Because a low-fat diet is abundant in carbohydrates, your body will retain excess carbohydrates as fat. Your metabolism will change from one that stores fat to one that burns it with the help of the successful Atkins diet. High-carb diets cause blood sugar levels to rise, which prompts the body to release more insulin. As a result, your body stores more fat and has a metabolism that burns sugar. Foods that are known to increase insulin and blood sugar are restricted on the Atkins diet. When you consume less carbs, your body is forced to burn fat instead of sugar for energy.

The original Atkins method, now known as Atkins 20®, is a four-phase program that begins with induction and aims to achieve 20 grams of net carbohydrates per day. Furthermore, Atkins has made the decision to provide Atkins 40®, a more flexible and extensive menu option.

As you approach your target weight on the Atkins 40® diet, you gradually increase your daily Net Carbohydrate intake from 40 grams, all the while burning fat for energy. In summary, Atkins 40 provides you with the flexibility to choose from a wide range of foods, including whole grains, legumes, fruits, nuts and seeds, vegetables, dairy products like whole Greek yogurt and cheeses, and whole grains. Atkins 40 places a strong emphasis on nutrient-dense carbs and portion management. Sugar additions are still discouraged.

Before you leap to Atkins 40, take into account the following factors so that you may choose the strategy that is most effective for you:

Continue using Atkins 20® if

- You need to shed almost forty pounds.
- You have diabetes or are pre-diabetic.

For males, your waist circumference is more than 40 inches, and for women, it is 35 inches.

You are happy with the progressive reintroduction of food options in a predetermined sequence.

Atkins 20 is giving you good results; as they say, "If it ain't broke, don't fix it!"

For Atkins 40®, switch if:

- You need to shed fewer than forty pounds.
- You do not have diabetes or pre-diabetes.
- You are fewer than 40 inches (35 inches for women) around the waist.
- You are breastfeeding a baby or expecting one.

As you're on Atkins 20, you're hoping for more variety in your diet.

What more is important to know about Atkins 40® is as follows:

Every day, you possess:

- About 15 grams of Net Carbs from Foundation Vegetables strong in fiber
- The remaining 25 grams of net carbohydrates are available for selection from the extended list of permitted foods, which includes whole grains, legumes, nuts, fruit, and Greek yogurt.
- a serving or two of six ounces of lean protein
- two to four meals a day that are high in healthful fats
- eight to nine glasses of water
- Taking a multivitamin every day

Chapter 2: Getting Started: Preparing for Success

You may start using Atkins and remain on track by paying attention to these 16 pointers:

Recognize what you are consuming and how the Atkins diet works. The core of Atkins is healthy eating. You'll discover which meals your body need to either gain or retain weight, as well as how to read nutrition labels, cut down on added sugar and other empty carbohydrates, and much more.

Atkins made just for you. Atkins offers two different plans that you may follow, depending on how much weight you need to lose: Atkins 20, which is the original plan and calls for ingesting 20 Net Carbs per day, or Atkins 40, which calls for consuming 40 grams of Net Carbs per day along with a wide variety of food alternatives.

Calculate your carbohydrates. Learn about Net Carbs and how to compute them by utilizing the helpful Carb Counter along with the lists of Acceptable Foods for your plan.

Be reasonable about portions—not compulsive. While using an Atkins diet doesn't require counting calories, you should still apply common sense. It should go without saying that consuming too many calories will slow down weight loss, while consuming too little calories can slow down your metabolism and impede weight reduction. Calorie concerns arise only if, even after strictly adhering to Atkins guidelines, weight loss remains unattainable. You may need to experiment with the following calorie ranges in order to lose weight, depending on your height, age, and metabolism: Men should limit their daily calorie intake to 1,800–2,200, while women should limit their daily calorie intake to 1,500–1,800.

Consume food often. That's correct—no famine! Eat two snacks and three regular-sized meals a day, regardless of the phase you're in. Alternatively, if you'd like, spread out your meals across four or five little ones. Consuming food every few hours helps you regulate your appetite and maintain stable blood sugar and energy levels. Eat till you're full but not overfull. Atkins offers a wide variety of items that make staying on track practical and simple, such as frozen meals, smoothies, snacks, and treats.

Add protein to each and every meal. Make sure your breakfast, lunch, and supper include four to six ounces of protein. Tall guys are allowed up to 8 ounces. Eggs, lean or fatty meat, poultry, and even beef cuts with marbling are acceptable options. Make careful to use enough olive oil or other healthy oils on salads and cooked vegetables when using leaner cuts.

Savor the natural fats in your meals. You eat less because fat makes food taste better and fills you up. Dietary fat is, in fact, essential to both general health and the Atkins diet. All fats are a healthy component of the Atkins diet, with the exception of synthetic trans fats (partially or fully hydrogenated oils).

Avoid sugar additions. Numerous foods and beverages, including most soft drinks, include added sugar in one of its various forms. They are all devoid of other nutrients and heavy in calories and carbohydrates. Alternatively, use non-caloric sweeteners (xylitol, stevia, or sucralose, which is sold as SplendaTM) to sweeten drinks. Don't exceed three packets per day; count each packet as one gram of net carbohydrates.

Consume vegetables. Make sure you receive your fill of 12 to 15 grams of carbs each day from Foundation Vegetables. You will immediately fulfill the USDA's recommendation to eat at least five servings of veggies each day. Along with lots of regularity, you'll also be receiving enough of fiber, which is important for controlling blood sugar. with addition to making you feel full, fiber aids with weight management.

Savor meals wherever you are—at home or at a restaurant. With Atkins, eating tasty natural foods is the main focus, as opposed to other diets that force people to buy pricey, pre-packaged meals or induce a phobia of eating. You'll discover how to make healthy meal choices whether you're eating home or out, traveling for work or pleasure, or dining at an ethnic restaurant or fast food joint. You'll quickly learn how to make wise decisions and maintain your course.

Cheers to that. In addition to being healthful, water and other liquids like tea and coffee (in moderation) help your body release water weight. Eight 8-ounce glasses should be consumed daily.

Consume vitamins on a daily basis. Supplementation is an excellent regimen for any weight reduction program when combined with a whole-foods diet. Unless you are iron deficient, take a daily multivitamin that contains minerals like potassium, magnesium, and calcium but not iron. Omega-3s are also an effective therapeutic agent whether taken as fish oil or another option.

Get in motion. Exercise and physical activity are a great complement to a balanced diet, with many advantages. Swimming, brisk walking, and other enjoyable activities are essential parts of the Atkins diet. Additionally, you will burn more calories as you gain muscle. It may be best to hold off on starting a new exercise routine or to intensify your current one for a few weeks after beginning an Atkins diet. Additionally, you may want to start out lightly with water aerobics or quick walks if you need to drop a lot of weight.

Monitor your accomplishments. We are discussing both weight and health metrics. Once a week, weigh and measure yourself at the hips, waist, and chest. Additionally, record your water and food consumption, as well as your successes and setbacks, in a notebook. Several studies show that those who maintain journals are better at controlling their weight than people who don't. Obtain baseline testing before to beginning the Atkins diet, then follow up on your lipid levels three to six months later. Get ready to be astounded by how much healthier they have grown.

Ask your friends and relatives for assistance. Inform the individuals who matter most in your life about their well-being. The highs and lows of their journey may be discussed with an Atkins friend. Don't forget to sign up for the Atkins.com Community Forum.
Make advance plans. Make sure you have the proper snacks and meals in your kitchen. Plan your meals in advance of going grocery shopping to avoid reverting to your previous, high-carbohydrate eating habits.

Chapter 3: Breakfast Recipes

Fennel, Carrot and Turkey Hash Recipe

Prep Time	Cook Time	Phase	SERVING	Protein	Fat	Fiber	Calories
10 Minutes	20 Minutes	Phase 3	1	18.1g	5.2g	1.5g	141.6cal

INGREDIENTS

1/3 tablespoon Canola Vegetable Oil
1 ounce Fennel Bulk
1/8 cup chopped Carrots
1/2 teaspoon Orange Zest
1/16 cup Freshly Squeezed Orange Juice
1/16 teaspoon Fennel Seed
1/4 tablespoon Tamari Soybean Sauce
1/8 cup chopped Scallions or Spring Onions
2 ounces Turkey Breast Meat (Fryer-Roasters, Cooked, Roasted)

DIRECTIONS

Chop the carrot and fennel. In a big pan, heat the oil over medium heat. Add the carrot and fennel and sauté for around three minutes. Juice and zest the orange.

Pour in the orange juice and zest. Simmer for approximately 4 minutes, or until liquid is practically absorbed.

Add the diced turkey, scallions, tamari, and fennel seeds. Cook until the turkey is well heated, about 6 more minutes. If desired, place a poached egg on top of each plate; each serving should include 1.3g of NC.

Leek Quiche Recipe

Net Carbs	Prep Time	Cook Time	SERVINGS	Phase	Protein	Fat	Calories
19.7g	15 Minutes	45 Min	6	Phase 3	22.2g	35.5g	490.2cal

INGREDIENTS

8 servings Atkins Pie Crust
1 tablespoon Unsalted Butter Stick
1 1/2 pounds Leeks
1/2 cup Heavy Cream
3 large Eggs (Whole)
1/2 teaspoon Salt
1/4 teaspoon Black Pepper
1 cup shredded Gruyere Cheese

DIRECTIONS

Set the oven to 350°F. Melt butter in a medium pan over medium heat. Add the chopped leeks and cook for 5 to 6 minutes, stirring now and again, until they become tender. Remove from the stove and stir in the cream. Give it five minutes.

Meanwhile, mix the eggs with the salt and pepper in a medium-sized basin. Mix the cream and leeks with the egg mixture. Cover the bottom of the pie shell with ¾ cup of cheese.

Spoon egg mixture into pie crust that has been prepared beforehand; top with remaining cheese. Bake for 45 minutes, or until the top is golden and the center is just set. If needed, activate the broiler and broil for 6 minutes from element 2, or until the top begins to brown.

Vegan Keto Coconut Protein Shake Recipe

Net Carbs	Prep Time	Cook Time	Phase	SERVING	Protein	Fat	Fiber	Calories
1.3g	5 Min	0 Min	Phase 1	1	24.4g	5.6g	1g	158.7cal

INGREDIENTS

1 cup Coconut Milk Unsweetened
1 ounce Protein Technologies International ProPlus Soy Protein Isolate
1/2 teaspoon Vanilla Extract

DIRECTIONS

For non-vegans or vegetarians, whey protein powder may be used instead; just add 1g NC to the total NC content.

In a blender, combine all ingredients and 2-4 ice cubes (depending on desired thickness). Think about substituting or adding coconut extract for the vanilla. Mix well and taste.

Breakfast Berry Parfait Recipe

Net Carbs	Prep Time	Cook Time	Phase	SERVINGS	Protein	Fat	Fiber	Calories
11.8g	15 Min	0 Min	Phase 2	4	10.3g	25.1g	7.8g	337.1cal

INGREDIENTS

2 cups Raspberries

1 1/2 cup, wholes Strawberries

Two and a half teaspoons of sucrose-based sweetener (sugar alternative)

1 cup Heavy Cream

1 tablespoon Vanilla Extract

6 ounces Greek Yogurt - Plain (Container)

1 bar Atkins Strawberry Shortcake Bar

DIRECTIONS

Blend 1 1/2 cups each of strawberries and raspberries in a blender with 1 1/2 teaspoons of sugar substitute.

Beat heavy cream, remaining 1 tablespoon sugar substitute, and vanilla in a large mixing bowl on medium speed with an electric mixer until soft peaks form. Beat in 1 1/2 single serving cartons of yogurt until stiff peaks form.

Make at least two layers of each of the berry mixture, cream filling, and crumbled Atkins bar in four parfait glasses.

Place a few of the leftover 1/2 cup raspberries on top of each before serving.

Keto Turkey Breakfast Meatloaf Recipe

Net Carbs	Prep Time	Cook Time	Phase	SERVINGS	Protein	Fat	Fiber	Calories
2.9g	15 Min	55 Min	Phase 1	8	38.8g	17.1g	2.4g	340.4cal

INGREDIENTS

1 10 oz package Frozen Chopped Spinach

Four medium-sized stalks, measuring between 7-1/2" and 8" in length Celery

1 medium (approx 2-3/4" long, 2-1/2" diameter) Sweet Red Peppers

24 ounce raw (yield after cooking) Turkey Breakfast Sausage

1 1/2 pounds Ground Turkey

6 large Eggs (Whole)

1 small Onion

1/2 tsp, ground Thyme (Dried)

1 medium (approx 2-3/4" long, 2-1/2" diameter) Green Sweet Pepper

1/8 teaspoon Nutmeg (Ground)

1/8 tablespoon Red or Cayenne Pepper

DIRECTIONS

Turn the oven on to 350°F.

After thawing, finely cut the spinach. Cut the bell peppers, white onion, and celery into dice.

Till well combined, add in the ground turkey sausage, celery, bell peppers, onion, and spinach.

Combine the eggs, nutmeg, thyme, cayenne, and 1/2 teaspoon of optional garlic powder. Add more salt and freshly ground black pepper to taste. Evenly distribute and transfer to two 4 x 9-inch standard quick bread pans.

Bake for 55 to 65 minutes, or until cooked through and browned on top. Serve right away or freeze for up to two months in individual servings.

Keto Scotch Eggs Recipe

Net Carbs	Prep Time	Cook Time	Phase	SERVINGS	Protein	Fat	Fiber	Calories
4.2g	20 Min	20 Min	Phase 1	4	33.5g	19.8g	5g	361.5cal

INGREDIENTS

8 large Boiled Eggs

1 large Egg (Whole)

1 teaspoon Tap Water

2 /4 cups Organic High Fiber Coconut Flour

12 ounce raw (yield after cooking) Turkey Breakfast Sausage

DIRECTIONS

Make sure the eggs are hard-boiled. Put one inch of cold water in a heavy pan and cover eight eggs. After bringing to a rolling boil, turn off the heat and let the eggs simmer for ten minutes. Remove the boiling water from the eggs right away and place them in a bath of ice water until they are cold enough to peel. After peeling the eggs, pat dry with a paper towel.

In a small bowl whisk together one egg and water. Put the coconut flour in another small bowl and, if like, season with salt and pepper. Put them both aside.

Form the sausage into eight equal balls. After that, flatten each ball into an oblong disk. Make care to uniformly cover the full surface of each egg as you wrap it around the sausage disk. Place each egg with a sausage cover on a platter.

In a big frying pan, heat up approximately 1 inch of oil over medium-high heat. After coating each egg completely, roll it in the whisked egg and then the coconut flour. Once the oil begins to shimmer, add all 8 eggs to the pan, being sure to leave at least 1/2 inch between each one if they fit. Fry for approximately 8 minutes on each side, or until golden brown on all sides. Then, using tongs, turn the food to the other side and continue cooking. After draining onto a paper towel, serve right away.

California Breakfast Burrito Recipe

Net Carbs	Prep Time	Cook Time	Phase	SERVINGS	Protein	Fat	Fiber	Calories
7.2g	20 Min	5 Min	Phase 2	4	22.2g	22.1g	5.8g	324.4cal

INGREDIENTS

1 serving Keto Tomatillo Salsa

4 tortillas Low Carb Tortillas

1 tablespoon Canola Vegetable Oil

3 large Scallions or Spring Onions

4 ounces Green Chili Peppers (Canned)

1 medium whole (2-3/5" diameter) Red Tomato

1/2 teaspoon Salt

1/4 teaspoon Black Pepper

8 large Eggs (Whole)

1/8 teaspoon Red or Cayenne Pepper

9 sprigs Cilantro (Coriander)

1/2 cup shredded Cheddar Cheese

DIRECTIONS

Preheat the oven to 325°F.

Tilt tortillas in foil and reheat for five to ten minutes.

Heat the oil in a medium-sized nonstick skillet over medium-high heat. Chop the tomatoes, chilies, and green onions. After adding them to the pan, season with pepper and salt. For three minutes, sauté.

Push mixture to the pan's side. Pour cayenne and eggs into the skillet. Simmer for a minute or two, stirring now and again with a rubber spatula, until soft, creamy curds start to develop.

Mix the veggie mixture with the eggs.

Spoon mixture into heated tortillas; top with 2 tablespoons cheese, 1 tablespoon salsa, and cilantro. Tortillas should be rolled.

Keto Sausage and Egg Muffin Cups Recipe

Net Carbs	Prep Time	Cook Time	Phase	SERVINGS	Protein	Fat	Fiber	Calories
2g	10 Min	30 Min	Phase 1	6	30.8g	32.8g	0.5g	436.8cal

INGREDIENTS

12 ounces Pork Italian Sausage
2/3 pound Ground Turkey
2/3 cup chopped Sweet Red Peppers
13 large Eggs (Whole)
1 tablespoon Parsley (Dried)
1/2 teaspoon Salt
1/4 teaspoon Black Pepper
1/4 teaspoon leaf Dried Thyme Leaves
1/4 teaspoon Paprika
1/8 teaspoon Nutmeg (Ground)
1/8 teaspoon Red or Cayenne Pepper

DIRECTIONS

Turn the oven on to 350°F. Muffin tin with twelve wells: grease it.

Sausage and ground turkey should be well combined.

Add one egg, diced red bell pepper, parsley, paprika, nutmeg, cayenne, salt, and pepper. Using your hands, combine all the ingredients and mix until well combined.

Evenly distribute the sausage mixture (approximately 66 grams per muffin well) across the 12 muffin wells. Making sure there are no holes in the mixture, press the sausage mixture up and slightly over the well rims to create an outer layer.

Place one egg into each well and pop them straight into the oven. Bake the eggs for 25 to 30 minutes, or until set. If you choose, top with cheese, salsa, or spicy sauce (don't forget to add the additional grams of NC!).

Keto French Toast Casserole Recipe

Net Carbs	Prep Time	Cook Time	Phase	SERVINGS	Protein	Fat	Fiber	Calories
5.4g	45 Min	80 Min	Phase 1	8	13.8g	36.7g	9.5g	449.5cal

INGREDIENTS

14 large Eggs (Whole)

3 tablespoons Xylitol

10 tablespoons Unsalted Butter Stick

1 cup Organic High Fiber Coconut Flour

1 1/2 teaspoons Baking Powder (Straight Phosphate, Double Acting)

3/4 teaspoon Salt

1 cup Heavy Cream

1 cup Coconut Milk Unsweetened

1 teaspoon Cinnamon

1/4 teaspoon Nutmeg (Ground)

1/2 cup Sugar Free Maple Flavored Syrup

DIRECTIONS

Turn the oven on to 350°F. Grease an 8 x 4-inch bread pan. Put aside.

In a medium bowl, whisk together 8 eggs, 1 tablespoon xylitol, and melted butter.
Blend the coconut flour, baking powder, and one-third teaspoon of salt using a sieve. Blend in the addition to the egg mixture until it thickens. Bake for 35 to 40 minutes, or until the edges become golden brown and peel away from the pan.

After letting it cool in the pan for ten minutes, move it to a wire rack and let it cool for a total of thirty minutes. If baking ahead of time, chill the baked goods and store them in the refrigerator for up to two weeks in an airtight container or zip-top bag. If used right away, cool completely, then break into

1-inch pieces and transfer to a small casserole dish or the same pan you used to bake the bread.

Mix six eggs, heavy cream, coconut milk (you may use water or soy milk in lieu of the coconut milk), two tablespoons xylitol, nutmeg, cinnamon, and a dash of salt in a medium-sized bowl. Cover the bread with the mixture and bake at 350°F for 50 minutes, or until the center is set. Divide into 8 portions and serve right away, covering each with 2 teaspoons of sugar-free pancake syrup (or roughly 1/3 cup for the whole dish).

Keto Zucchini Bread Muffins Recipe

Net Carbs	Prep Time	Cook Time	Phase	SERVINGS	Protein	Fat	Fiber	Calories
2.4g	10 Min	25 Min	Phase 1	6	10.3g	12.4g	5.9g	174.8cal

INGREDIENTS

2 large Eggs (Whole)

2 tablespoons Canola Vegetable Oil

1 teaspoon Vanilla Extract

4 1/2 ounces Zucchini

1 cup Organic 100% Whole Ground Golden Flaxseed Meal

1 ounce Vanilla Whey Protein

1/3 cup Sucralose Based Sweetener (Sugar Substitute)

1 1/2 teaspoons Cinnamon

3/4 teaspoon Baking Powder (Straight Phosphate, Double Acting)

1/4 teaspoon Salt

1/8 teaspoon Allspice Ground

1/8 teaspoon Nutmeg (Ground)

DIRECTIONS

Set oven temperature to 350°F. Grease six wells in a typical muffin tray that is non-stick.

Whisk the oil, vanilla, and eggs together in a small dish. Beat with a whisk until foamy, approximately one minute. Add the shredded zucchini to the bowl and stir everything together.

Stir in the protein powder, baking powder, granulated sugar replacement, flax meal, salt, and spices. Using a spoon, combine and mix.

Bake for twenty-five minutes, or until cooked through, golden, and slightly puffed. If preferred, enjoy it with cream cheese.

Cinnamon Crumb Coffee Cake Recipe

Net Carbs	Prep Time	Cook Time	Phase	SERVINGS	Protein	Fat	Fiber	Calories
11.4g	30 Min	40 Min	Phase 4	12	6.7g	34.7g	3.1g	383cal

INGREDIENTS

3/4 cup 100% Stone Ground Whole Wheat Pastry Flour
3/4 cup Whole Grain Soy Flour
1/2 cup Whole Wheat Flour
1 teaspoon Baking Powder (Straight Phosphate, Double Acting)
1 teaspoon Baking Soda
1/2 teaspoon Salt
2 large Eggs (Whole)
1 teaspoon Vanilla Extract
1 cup Sour Cream (Cultured)
1 1/4 cups Unsalted Butter Stick
2 cups Sucralose Based Sweetener (Sugar Substitute)
1/2 cup, dry, yield Oatmeal
1 1/2 cup, halves Pecan Nuts
2 teaspoons Cinnamon

DIRECTIONS

Turn the oven on to 350°F. Grease and put aside a 9 x 13-inch baking pan.

To make the cake, combine the whole-wheat flour, soy flour, pastry flour, baking soda, baking powder, and salt in a medium-sized basin. Whisk together the eggs, sour cream, and vanilla in a large liquid measuring cup until well blended.

Beat 1/2 cup butter and 1 cup sugar substitute in a large bowl on medium speed with an electric mixer until smooth and fluffy, approximately 4 minutes. Start and finish with the flour combination, then alternately add the egg mixture and flour mixture to the butter.

To make the topping, pulse the oats, 3/4 cup butter, pecans, sugar replacement, and cinnamon in a blender until a coarse meal-like texture is achieved.

Spread two thirds of the batter into the prepared pan in order to build the cake. To form pockets of topping within the batter, sprinkle half of the topping over the batter and gently swirl with a knife.

After spooning the remaining batter over the topping, evenly distribute the remaining topping. Bake for approximately 40 minutes, or until a knife inserted in the middle comes out clean. Cake is cooled in a pan resting on a wire rack. Heat or serve at room temperature. Yields twelve servings.

Mushroom Scramble Recipe

Net Carbs	Prep Time	Cook Time	Phase	SERVINGS	Protein	Fat	Fiber	Calories
4g	10 Min	6 Min	Phase 1	6	11.7g	14.2g	0.8g	192.9cal

INGREDIENTS

1 cup Mushroom Pieces and Stems
1/2 cup chopped Onions
3 tablespoons Extra Virgin Olive Oil
14 ounces Firm Silken Tofu
1 cup Baby Spinach
1/4 cup shredded Cheddar Cheese
3 tablespoons Parmesan Cheese (Grated)
4 large Eggs (Whole)
1/8 teaspoon leaf Dried Thyme Leaves
8 Cherry Tomatoes

DIRECTIONS

Cook the white onion and mushrooms in the oil in a big, nonstick pan over medium-high heat until they are tender, approximately 3 minutes.

Cook for a further three minutes after adding the tofu and spinach.

Cook until the egg is set, stirring in the tomatoes, eggs, Parmesan, and Cheddar cheeses along with 1/8 tsp thyme.

Serve right away.

Keto Mini Chocolate Chip Muffins Recipe

Net Carbs	Prep Time	Cook Time	Phase	SERVINGS	Protein	Fat	Fiber	Calories
2.7g	10 Min	15 Min	Phase 2	24	1.7g	5.2g	2.1g	64.7cal

INGREDIENTS

2/3 cup Almond Flour, Blanched

1/2 cup Sucralose Based Sweetener (Sugar Substitute)

1/3 cup Coconut Flour

1 teaspoon Baking Powder (Straight Phosphate, Double Acting)

3/4 teaspoon Xanthan Gum

1/4 teaspoon Salt

1/2 cup Sour Cream (Cultured)

2 tablespoons Unsalted Butter Stick

2 tablespoons Heavy Cream

1 fluid ounce Tap Water

2 teaspoons Vanilla Extract

4 ounces Lily's Sugar Free Chocolate Chips

DIRECTIONS

Preheat the oven to 350°F. 24 small muffin wells should be greased or lined with paper liners.

Almond flour, sugar replacement, coconut flour, xanthan gum, baking powder, and salt should all be combined in a bowl.

Combine the sour cream, heavy cream, melted butter, water, and vanilla in a separate dish and mix them together.

To the flour mixture, add the sour cream mixture. Mix well until fully incorporated. Add chocolate chips and fold.

Evenly fill muffin wells, about 1 tablespoon each muffin. Bake for 20 minutes, or until a toothpick inserted in the middle comes out clean and top is gently browned.

After five minutes of cooling in the pans, remove the muffins and let them cool fully on wire racks.

Keto Crustless Spinach Quiche Recipe

Net Carbs	Prep Time	Cook Time	Phase	SERVINGS	Protein	Fat	Fiber	Calories
3.6g	20 Min	30 Min	Phase 1	4	16.1g	38.1g	2.1g	427.3cal

INGREDIENTS

2 teaspoons Canola Vegetable Oil
1/2 cup chopped Scallions or Spring Onions
6 1/2 ounces Frozen Chopped Spinach
4 large Eggs (Whole)
1 cup Heavy Cream
1 cup shredded Muenster Cheese
1/4 teaspoon Salt
1/4 teaspoon Black Pepper
1/8 teaspoon Nutmeg (Ground)

DIRECTIONS

Set oven temperature to 175°C/350°F. Grease a 9-inch pie tin very lightly.

Heat the oil in a large skillet over medium-high heat. Add onions and simmer until soft, stirring from time to time. Chop the frozen spinach and add it to the skillet. Cook the spinach until it becomes heated throughout and all of the moisture is gone.

Mix the eggs, cream, cheese, nutmeg, salt, and pepper in a big basin. Blend in the spinach mixture by stirring it in. Fill the pie pan with prepared filling.

Bake for approximately 30 minutes in a preheated oven, or until the eggs are set. Prior to serving, let cool for ten minutes.

Add chopped spinach or whole baby spinach to the skillet with the onions and a tablespoon of water if you're using fresh spinach. Cook for two cups at a time until the spinach starts to wilt, then add another cup. Continue cooking until

the spinach is completely wilted and the
moisture has evaporated before adding it
to the egg mixture.

Greek Easter Bread Recipe

Net Carbs	Prep Time	Cook Time	Phase	SERVINGS	Protein	Fat	Fiber	Calories
6.5g	20 Min	45 Min	Phase 2	12	18.2g	11.6g	2.9g	207.9cal

INGREDIENTS

4 large Eggs (Whole)

1 teaspoon Vinegar

1 packet (2.5 teaspoons) Active Dry Yeast

2 1/2 cups Whole Grain Soy Flour

4 ounces Vital Wheat Gluten

1 1/2 teaspoons Baking Powder (Sodium Aluminum Sulfate, Double Acting)

1/4 teaspoon Salt

4 tablespoons Butter

1 large Egg Yolk

1/4 cup Sucralose Based Sweetener (Sugar Substitute)

1 teaspoon Orange Zest

1/2 teaspoon Cinnamon

1/8 cup sliced Almonds

DIRECTIONS

For the eggs: Hard boil the eggs and then transfer them to a big enough stainless steel dish to stay in a single layer. Add 1 tablespoon red food coloring, 1 cup water, and vinegar and bring to a boil. Pour over eggs; leave for at least five minutes to let color seep into the egg shells. Take the eggs out of the dish and place them on a rack to dry.

Regarding bread: Use parchment paper to line a baking sheet. Sprinkle the yeast into 1/2 cup of warm water to activate it, then watch it froth. Put aside. In a large basin, combine soy flour, wheat gluten, baking powder, and salt. Combine one cup of warm water, yeast water, egg yolk, melted butter, sugar replacement, orange peel, and cinnamon. Blend with a spoon to create a soft dough after adding to the flour mixture. Knead manually for one minute. Shape the dough into a 6 × 8 rectangle and cut it into 3 lengthwise pieces. Each strip should be rolled into a 22–24-inch rope. Braide the strips, working straight onto the baking sheet. Form braid into circular shapes with a diameter of 10 to 12 inches.

Place eggs equally spaced along the braid. Place a plastic cover over it and let it rise for one to two hours, or until its mass has doubled.

About fifteen minutes before the dough is done rising, preheat the oven to 350°F. Lightly coat the dough with the leftover egg white (from the yolk) and scatter almonds on top.

Bake for 45 to 50 minutes, or until firm to the touch and golden brown. Take out of the oven and place on a wire rack to cool fully. Yields twelve servings.

Keto Eggs with Avocado and Tomato Recipe

Net Carbs	Prep Time	Cook Time	Phase	SERVING	Protein	Fat	Fiber	Calories
4g	5 Min	5 Min	Phase 1	1	14.8g	23.4g	6.6g	302.5cal

INGREDIENTS

2 large Eggs (Whole)
1/2 medium whole (2-3/5" diameter) Red Tomatoes
Half a fruit (no seeds and skin) that is a California avocado

DIRECTIONS

Cook an egg whatever you'd like.

Cut the avocado and tomato into slices.

Eggs, avocado, and tomato are layered. If desired, add some chopped green onions or paprika.

Almond Raspberry Smoothie Recipe

Net Carbs	Prep Time	Cook Time	Phase	SERVING	Protein	Fat	Fiber	Calories
10.3g	5 Min	0 Min	Phase 2	1	18.2g	13.7g	6.9g	259.4cal

INGREDIENTS

4 ounces Greek Yogurt - Plain (Container)
1/2 cup Red Raspberries
20 each wholes Blanched & Slivered Almonds
1/2 cup Pure Almond Milk - Unsweetened Original

DIRECTIONS

Feel free to experiment with other berries and nuts to make your own protein-rich smoothie. Make sure the frozen raspberries you use don't have any extra sugar.

In a blender, combine the yogurt, almond milk, raspberries, and almonds; process until smooth and creamy.

Keto Italian Frittata Recipe

Net Carbs	Prep Time	Cook Time	Phase	SERVINGS	Protein	Fat	Fiber	Calories
7g	20 Min	20 Min	Phase 1	4	25.1g	30.3g	1.3g	406.8cal

INGREDIENTS

1 tablespoon Light Olive Oil

1 tablespoon Unsalted Butter Stick

2 cloves Garlic

1/2 cup chopped Onions

1 large Zucchini

1 teaspoon leaf Basil (Dried)

8 ounce raw (yield after cooking) Italian Sausage

8 large Eggs (Whole)

2 tablespoons Tap Water

1/4 teaspoon Salt

1/4 teaspoon Black Pepper

1/3 cup Parmesan Cheese (Grated)

DIRECTIONS

Warm up the broiler.

In a large ovenproof skillet, heat the oil and butter over medium heat. Add the diced white onion and minced garlic to the pan, then sauté for two to three minutes, or until the ingredients are softened. Slicing the zucchini, add it to the pan with the basil and cook, turning regularly, for 5 to 6 minutes, or until the zucchini is tender but not limp. Cook the sausage for two to three minutes, stirring now and again.

In the meanwhile, mix the eggs, water, salt, and pepper in a large basin. Over the meat and vegetable combination, pour the egg mixture into the heated pan. Allow to cook, undisturbed, for a few seconds, then tilt the pan to allow the raw eggs to flow to the edges and use a spatula to slide the eggs into the center. For 4 to 5 minutes, or until the eggs are nearly set (the tops will still be wet), keep heating and stirring the egg mixture.

After adding the cheese and placing it under the broiler, wait two to three minutes, or until the eggs are cooked through and the cheese is bubbling.

Slice into quarters and serve right away.

Keto Sweet and Salty Almonds Recipe

Net Carbs	Prep Time	Cook Time	Phase	SERVINGS	Protein	Fat	Fiber	Calories
2g	5 Min	15 Min	Phase 2	16	4g	9.1g	2.3g	106.8cal

INGREDIENTS

1 large Egg White

1/3 cup Sucralose Based Sweetener (Sugar Substitute)

3/4 dash Salt

2 teaspoons Cinnamon

2 cup, wholes Almonds

DIRECTIONS

Preheat the oven to 350°F.

In a larger bowl, mix together the egg white, sugar substitute, cinnamon, and salt. Using a fork, beat until foamy. Toss in almonds to coat. Spread out on a baking sheet covered with aluminum foil or a nonstick baking sheet in a single layer.

Bake, rotating once, for 12 to 15 minutes, or until toasted and crisp. After taking out of the oven, put the baking sheet on a cooling rack. After the nuts have cooled, take them out of the pan and keep them for up to a week at room temperature in an airtight container.

Keto Crustless Broccoli Quiche Recipe

Net Carbs	Prep Time	Cook Time	Phase	SERVINGS	Protein	Fat	Fiber	Calories
6.8g	15 Min	60 Min	Phase 1	6	12.4g	15.2g	0.2g	208.5cal

INGREDIENTS

1 teaspoon Extra Virgin Olive Oil

1/4 cup White Onion, raw, chopped

4 large Eggs (Whole)

1 cup Half and Half Cream

1 cup shredded Cheddar Cheese

1/2 cup Tap Water

1/4 teaspoon Thyme

1/4 teaspoon leaf Oregano

1/2 teaspoon Salt

1/4 teaspoon Black Pepper

1/4 teaspoon Rosemary (Dried)

1 pound Broccoli Flower Clusters

DIRECTIONS

Turn the oven on to 375°F.

Coat a pie dish, measuring 9 or 10 inches, with virgin olive oil.

The oil should be heated to medium-high heat in a small skillet. Add the chopped white onion and simmer for approximately 3 minutes, or until softened. Move to a medium-sized bowl and let it cool.

Lightly whisk eggs into onion mixture. Blend in half-and-half, a half-cup of cheese, water, oregano, thyme, salt, pepper, and rosemary.

Add broccoli to the bottom of the pie pan. Cover with egg mixture and top with remaining 1/2 cup cheese.

Bake for 50 to 60 minutes, or until a knife inserted in the center comes out clean and the quiche is golden brown. Or instead bake them for 15 to 20 minutes, or until completely set, in a muffin tray that has been buttered. They're a convenient supper or snack for on-the-go.

Chocolate Pancakes Recipe

Net Carbs	Prep Time	Cook Time	Phase	SERVINGS	Protein	Fat	Fiber	Calories
10.3g	10 Min	5 Min	Phase 2	4	15.2g	19g	3.9g	280.6cal

INGREDIENTS

1 cup Whole Grain Soy Flour
2 tablespoons Cocoa Powder (Unsweetened)
6 tablespoons Sucralose Based Sweetener (Sugar Substitute)
1/2 teaspoon Baking Powder (Straight Phosphate, Double Acting)
1/4 teaspoon Salt
3/4 cup Whole Milk
2 large Eggs (Whole)
3 tablespoons Unsalted Butter Stick
2 teaspoons Vanilla Extract

DIRECTIONS

Mix sugar replacement, baking powder, cocoa powder, and salt with soy flour. Mix until smooth after adding the milk, eggs, melted butter, and extract. Let the batter settle for five minutes.

Apply a thin layer of cooking spray to a big nonstick skillet and heat it over medium heat. For each pancake, use two teaspoons of batter. Cook for 3–4 minutes, or until little bubbles start to form around the edges; turn and cook for an additional 30–45 seconds.

Chapter 4: Lunch Recipes

Roast Beef, Red Bell Pepper and Provolone Lettuce Wraps Recipe

Net Carbs	Prep Time	Cook Time	Phase	SERVING	Protein	Fat	Fiber	Calories
2.7g	5 Min	0 Min	Phase 1	1	44.5g	44.9g	1g	603.5cal

INGREDIENTS

2 inner leaves Romaine Lettuce (salad)

2 ounces Provolone Cheese

1 tablespoon Real Mayonnaise

1/2 teaspoon Horseradish

4 ounces boneless, cooked Roast Beef

1/4 medium (approx 2-3/4" long, 2-1/2" diameter) Red Sweet Pepper

DIRECTIONS

Take off the lettuce leaves' bottoms. Place flat on a sanitized surface. Top each with a slice of cheese.

Mix the horseradish and mayonnaise together, add optional garlic powder, season with salt and freshly ground black pepper. Apply to slices of cheese. Add a layer of roast meat after that.

Trim and thinly slice the red bell pepper, then arrange it on one end of the roast beef, cheese, and lettuce. Beginning where you arranged the pepper strips, roll up until the roll is completely folded up. Use a toothpick to secure, then repeat for the second roll-up and consume right away.

Bacon-Egg Salad Flatout Wrap Recipe

Net Carbs	Prep Time	Cook Time	Phase	SERVING	Protein	Fat	Fiber	Calories
8.6g	10 Min	0 Min	Phase 3	1	34.2g	33.9g	8.3g	497.5cal

INGREDIENTS

2 large Boiled Eggs

1 tablespoon Real Mayonnaise

1/2 tsp or 1 packet Yellow Mustard

1 flatbread Light Original Flatbread

1 1/2 oz, cookeds Turkey Bacon

1 inner leaf Romaine Lettuce (salad)

DIRECTIONS

Combine chopped eggs, mustard, and mayonnaise. Taste and adjust with extra salt and pepper.

After the lettuce has been smoothed out on one rounded end of the Flatout, spread mixture over it. Crumble cooked bacon over top, fold up, and cut in half.

Buffalo Chicken Salad Recipe

Net Carbs	Prep Time	Cook Time	Phase	SERVINGS	Protein	Fat	Fiber	Calories
9.7g	0 Min	45 Min	Phase 2	2	27.2g	71.1g	9.1g	814.6cal

INGREDIENTS

1/2 fruit (2-1/8" diameter) Lemon

1 medium (4-1/8" long) Young Green Onions

1/4 cup Real Mayonnaise

2 tablespoons Sour Cream

2/3 ounce Blue Cheese

1/8 teaspoon Garlic Powder

1 head Cos or Romaine Lettuce

2 stalk, medium (7-1/2" - 8" long) Celery

1 medium (approx 2-3/4" long, 2-1/2" diameter) Red Sweet Pepper

1 medium Tomato

1 large Egg

5 1/3 tablespoons Apple Cider Vinegar

1/4 cup Olive Oil

1/3 teaspoon Salt

1/4 teaspoon Black Pepper

1/8 teaspoon Celery Salt

1/8 teaspoon Red or Cayenne Pepper

2 thigh, bone removeds Chicken Thigh Meat and Skin (Broilers or Fryers)

DIRECTIONS

Set aside a sheet pan and preheat the oven to 450°.

Juice the lemon and scrape out the seeds into a big dish. Chop the onions finely and add them to the lemon juice together with the sour cream, blue cheese, mayonnaise, and garlic powder. Stir to mix and put away.

Prepare the veggies by dicing the tomato into 1-inch pieces, slicing the red pepper into ¼-inch strips, cutting the romaine lettuce into 1-inch pieces, and chopping the celery into ½-inch slices on the bias. Refrigerate until required, then combine all the veggies in the big bowl with the dressing (do not stir).

Use a fork to whisk the egg in a medium-sized bowl. Whisk in the cayenne pepper, celery salt, apple cider vinegar, olive oil, and salt and pepper until well mixed and foamy.

After using a paper towel to pat dry each chicken thigh, dip it into the egg mixture and transfer it to the prepared sheet pan. Bake for 18 to 20 minutes, rotating the thighs and coating them with the egg mixture many times, or until they are crisp and cooked through. Slice the chicken into halves or quarters.

Take the salad out of the fridge, mix the veggies with the dressing, and then portion it onto two plates. Place half of the chicken on top of each platter and serve.

Cheese Straws Recipe

Net Carbs	Prep Time	Cook Time	Phase	SERVINGS	Protein	Fat	Fiber	Calories
1.7g	150 Min	12 Min	Phase 2	13	7.2g	10.1g	0.9g	127.4cal

INGREDIENTS

1 serving Atkins Soy-Free Flour Mix
6 tablespoons Unsalted Butter Stick
1/2 teaspoon Garlic Powder
3/4 cup shredded Cheddar Cheese
1/4 cup Parmesan Cheese (Grated)
2 large Eggs (Whole)
1/2 serving Garlic Salt

DIRECTIONS

To prepare the Atkins Soy-Free Flour Mix for this dish, use the Atkins instructions. One cup will be required.

In a food processor, combine the baking mix, butter, and garlic powder. Mix until mixture has the consistency of coarse crumbs. Add the eggs and cheese. Just until the dough comes together, pulse.

Place the dough onto a large parchment paper sheet. Shape gently into a round, flat shape. Cover dough with a second piece of parchment. Roll or press the dough into a rectangle about 6 by 12 and approximately 1/2 thick. Put in a resealable bag and chill for at least two hours (or overnight) to make sure it becomes very solid.

Preheat the oven to 375°F.

Roll out the dough horizontally on the counter. Take off the dough's top parchment layer. Add a pinch of garlic salt and gently press it into the dough. Cut the dough into forty 6-inch-long strips using a sharp knife. Stretch the strips out onto a baking sheet without oil. Bake for 11 to 13 minutes, or until gently browned, keeping a watchful eye out for burning during the final 5 minutes. Straws may be slid onto a cooling rack. Store in an airtight jar until cooled. One dish is equivalent to three sticks.

Ham, Cream Cheese and Dill Pickle Roll-Ups Recipe

Net Carbs	Prep Time	Cook Time	Phase	SERVING	Protein	Fat	Fiber	Calories
2.5g	5 Min	0 Min	Phase 1	1	17.7g	20.2g	0.7g	266.2cal

INGREDIENTS

2 ounces boneless, cooked Fresh Ham
2 tablespoons Cream Cheese
2 spears Pickles

DIRECTIONS

For every 1-ounce piece of ham, spread 1 tablespoon of cream cheese. Each ham slice should have a pickle spear at one end before being rolled up. If preferred, use a toothpick to secure it.

Keto Garlic Ranch Dressing Recipe

Net Carbs	Prep Time	Cook Time	Phase	SERVINGS	Protein	Fat	Fiber	Calories
0.9g	20 Min	0 Min	Phase 1	10	0.6g	12.3g	0g	116.2cal

INGREDIENTS

3/4 cup Real Mayonnaise

1/2 cup Buttermilk (Reduced Fat, Cultured)

3/4 teaspoon Onion Powder

2 tablespoons Parsley

1/2 teaspoon Garlic

1 teaspoon Dijon Mustard

1/8 teaspoon Salt

1/8 teaspoon Black Pepper

1 teaspoon Fresh Lemon Juice

DIRECTIONS

In a blender, combine all ingredients and purée until smooth. Taste and adjust with salt and freshly ground black pepper. Yields: 10 portions, using 2 tablespoons in each serving.

Keto Crab and Avocado Salad Recipe

Net Carbs	Prep Time	Cook Time	Phase	SERVINGS	Protein	Fat	Fiber	Calories
2.2g	20 Min	0 Min	Phase 1	4	22.1g	15.9g	4g	251.7cal

INGREDIENTS

3 tablespoons mayonnaise, real

2 tablespoons lime juice, 100%, fresh squeezed

1/2 teaspoon cumin seeds

1/4 teaspoon paprika

1/4 teaspoon table salt

1/4 teaspoon black pepper, ground

16 ounces canned crab

2 eas fresh celery stalk, medium, 7 1/2" to 8"

1 ea fresh avocado

3 cups fresh watercress, chopped

DIRECTIONS

Combine mayonnaise, lime juice, paprika, cumin, salt, and pepper in a medium-sized bowl.
]
Add chopped celery and drained crab meat. Till the coating is uniform, fold together. If desired, add salt and pepper after tasting.

Cut the avocado into cubes and incorporate it gently into the mixture.

Alternatively, instead of chopping the avocado, just remove the seed and shell; this salad looks fantastic served in the well of the avocado halves.

Arrange the watercress in four equal portions; cover with about one cup of salad on each dish.

Please wait, Your Review is Very Important…

Dear Reader,

I hope this message finds you well. Thank you for choosing to read the Atkins Diet Book for Beginners 2024. Your feedback is incredibly valuable to me, and I would love to hear your thoughts on the book. Whether you've just started, are halfway through, or have finished reading, your perspective matters.

Your feedback is immensely appreciated and will help me enhance future works.

Thank you for taking the time to share your thoughts on the Atkins Diet Book for Beginners 2024. I appreciate your help very much.

Happy reading!

Dr. Valerie Kennedy

Chapter 5: Dinner Recipes

Maehing's Chicken Eggplant Casserole Recipe

Net Carbs	Prep Time	Cook Time	Phase	SERVINGS	Protein	Fat	Fiber	Calories
5.5g	40 Min	35 Min	Phase 3	8	37.8g	20.7g	6.4g	383.3cal

INGREDIENTS

2 servings Atkins Low Carb Wheat Bread

3 eggplant, peeled (yield from 1-1/4 lb) Eggplant

3/4 teaspoon Salt

1/3 cup Parmesan Cheese (Grated)

1 cup shredded Cheddar Cheese

Four medium-sized (4-1/8-inch-long) spring onions

1/3 cup Cilantro (Coriander)

3 large Eggs (Whole)

3 tablespoons Unsalted Butter Stick

3 tablespoons Sour Cream (Cultured)

24 ounces boneless, cooked Chicken Breast

1/2 teaspoon Paprika

DIRECTIONS

Preheat the oven to 350°F. Apply nonstick cooking spray to a 9 x 13-inch baking pan and put it aside.

Boil eggplant in gently salted water for 15 minutes with a half cover on until it becomes soft. After draining, pat dry. Chop the chicken and reserve.

The bread should be processed into tiny crumbs in the bowl of a food processor with a metal blade (or a four-sided box grater). Pulse to mix in the Parmesan cheese.

Mash the eggplant slightly in a big dish. Stir in half of the breadcrumb mixture, eggs, butter, sour cream, green onions, cilantro, and salt and pepper. Add the chopped chicken and fold.

Pour mixture into a pan that has been prepared. Spatula to smooth top. Add paprika and the remaining breadcrumb mixture on top. Bake for thirty-five minutes. Allow to stand for five minutes before serving.

Keto Steaks with Green Onion and Caper Sauce Recipe

Net Carbs	Prep Time	Cook Time	Phase	SERVINGS	Protein	Fat	Fiber	Calories
0.8g	10 Min	8 Min	Phase 2	4	49.6g	28.9g	0.7g	474.7cal

INGREDIENTS

2 large Scallions or Spring Onions
4 tablespoons drained Capers
3 teaspoons Dijon Mustard
1 tablespoon Red Wine Vinegar
1/4 cup Extra Virgin Olive Oil
2 tablespoons Parsley
24 ounces Rib Eye Steak

DIRECTIONS

Set the broiler pan to 4 inches from the heat source and preheat the broiler.

Use salt and pepper to season the steaks, then cook them for the desired doneness (medium-rare is about 3 to 4 minutes each side).

As the steaks cook, make the sauce: Mix the mustard, onions, capers, and red wine vinegar together in a small bowl. Drizzle in olive oil gradually and mix until a small thickening occurs. Add the parsley and season with salt and pepper to taste.

When serving, spoon sauce over the steaks.

Keto Chili-Beef Kebabs Recipe

Net Carbs	Prep Time	Cook Time	Phase	SERVINGS	Protein	Fat	Fiber	Calories
1.3g	30 Min	12 Min	Phase 1	8	23.1g	19.9g	0.8g	283.4cal

INGREDIENTS

2 tablespoons Canola Vegetable Oil
3 teaspoons Garlic
1 tablespoon Chili Powder
1 teaspoon Salt
1/8 teaspoon Red or Cayenne Pepper
2 pounds Beef Top Sirloin (Trimmed to 1/8" Fat, Choice Grade)
8 medium (4-1/8" long) Scallions or Spring Onions
2 tablespoons Parsley

DIRECTIONS

In a bowl, mix together oil, minced garlic, chili powder, salt, and red pepper. To coat, add the meat tossing. Let it marinate for one hour.

If used, soak bamboo skewers in water fifteen minutes before cooking, then heat your grill to medium.

Alternatively, skewer chunks of meat and half green onions. Kebabs should be cooked through after 10 to 15 minutes of grilling, flipping them regularly. After adding parsley, serve.

Beef Sauteed with Vegetables Over Romaine Recipe

Net Carbs	Prep Time	Cook Time	Phase	SERVINGS	Protein	Fat	Fiber	Calories
7.6g	10 Min	35 Min	Phase 1	6	28.6g	32.5g	2.7g	446.6cal

INGREDIENTS

1 1/2 pounds Ground Beef (80% Lean / 20% Fat)

1/4 cup chopped Onions

1/4 cup chopped Green Sweet Pepper

15 ounces Tomato Sauce (Canned)

4 tablespoons Tomato Paste

3 teaspoons Sucralose Based Sweetener (Sugar Substitute)

6 cups shredded Cos or Romaine Lettuce

6 ounces Cheddar Cheese

DIRECTIONS

In a nonstick pan over medium-high heat, brown the meat. In the last five minutes of browning, add the peppers and onions.

After removing any surplus fat from the pan, mix in the tomato paste, tomato sauce, and sugar replacement. Season with freshly ground black pepper and salt. Simmer for 30 minutes at a low temperature.

Serve right now over Cheddar-topped shredded Romaine.

Keto Garlic Shrimp with Avocado Dip Recipe

Net Carbs	Prep Time	Cook Time	Phase	SERVINGS	Protein	Fat	Fiber	Calories
1.4g	15 Min	5 Min	Phase 1	8	8.4g	9.7g	3.4g	134.6cal

INGREDIENTS

2 eas fresh avocado

1 Jalapeno Pepper

1/2 teaspoon Salt

48 medium Shrimps

1 tablespoon Extra Virgin Olive Oil

1 teaspoon Garlic

1/8 teaspoon Red or Cayenne Pepper

DIRECTIONS

Halve the avocado, remove the pit, and scrape the flesh into a food processor to make a dip. Take off the jalapeño's stem and seeds, reserving some for a spicier dip. Blend the blend until it's smooth, then add optional salt and freshly ground black pepper for seasoning. Alternatively, purée without the jalapeño and use three tablespoons of spicy sauce. Put aside. Grill over medium-high heat before using.

Shrimp should be rubbed with oil, chopped garlic, cayenne, and salt in a bowl. Leave tiny gaps between each of the eight skewers as you thread three prawns onto them. (To prevent burning, soak wooden skewers in water for an hour before using.)

Shrimp should be cooked through and golden after 2 and a half minutes of covered grilling. Accompany with avocado dip.

Keto Spice-Rubbed Lamb Loins with Cucumber Salad Recipe

Net Carbs	Prep Time	Cook Time	Phase	SERVINGS	Protein	Fat	Fiber	Calories
6.6g	25 Min	120 Min	Phase 2	4	33.1g	31.4g	2.3g	453.7cal

INGREDIENTS

1 1/2 tablespoons Coriander Seed

1 tablespoon Onion Powder

1 tablespoon Garlic Powder

1 tablespoon Cumin

1 teaspoon Chili Powder

2 teaspoons Turmeric (Ground)

1 teaspoon Nutmeg (Ground)

24 ounce boneless, raw (yield after cooking) Lamb

2 cup, pared, choppeds Cucumber (Peeled)

1/4 cup (8 fluid ounces) Plain Yogurt (Whole Milk)

1 tablespoon chopped Scallions or Spring Onions

1 serving Coconut Milk

2 tablespoons Tap Water

DIRECTIONS

Combine the coriander, cumin, chili powder, onion powder, garlic powder, turmeric, nutmeg, salt, and black pepper in a small bowl.

After removing any surplus fat from the lamb medallions, coat them with the spice blend. Allow the ingredients to marinate in a 9-by-13-inch baking dish for a minimum of two hours, but no more than overnight.

Make the salad in the meanwhile. Combine the cucumber, yogurt, and scallions in a medium-sized bowl. Store in the refrigerator until ready to serve.

Heat the canola oil in a cast-iron pan over medium-high heat. After removing the medallions from the marinade, grill them for two to three minutes on each side, or until done. Take it out of the pan, let it cool for five minutes, and then add some salt and pepper to taste. Remove any leftover spices and lamb pieces from the skillet and discard any extra oil in the pan.

In the meanwhile, mix the water and coconut milk together in a small dish. Scrape the spices and lamb fragments off the skillet's bottom and sides with a spatula. Stir in the pan scrapings and add the coconut milk mixture. Bring to a boil while stirring.

Arrange a quarter of the cucumber salad on each dish for serving. Arrange a lamb medallion next to every salad and cover one with a quarter of the coconut sauce.

White Pizza with Broccoli Recipe

Net Carbs	Prep Time	Cook Time	Phase	SERVINGS	Protein	Fat	Fiber	Calories
12.1g	10 Min	10 Min	Phase 3	8	30.2g	21.8g	5.6g	372.8cal

INGREDIENTS

1 package Bakers Yeast (Active Dry)

1 1/2 cups (8 fluid ounces) Water

2 1/2 cups Whole Grain Soy Flour

4 ounces Vital Wheat Gluten

1 1/2 teaspoons Baking Powder (Sodium Aluminum Sulfate, Double Acting)

1/4 teaspoon Salt

5 tablespoons Olive Oil

2 cloves Garlic

1 pound Broccoli

3/4 cup Ricotta Cheese (Whole Milk)

1/2 cup shredded Mozzarella Cheese (Whole Milk)

4 tablespoons Parmesan Cheese (Grated)

1 teaspoon Oregano

DIRECTIONS

Lightly spray a 14-inch pizza pan with air holes with oil to prepare it. Put aside. In a small basin, mix yeast with 1/2 cup warm water. Let it bubble for a few minutes by setting it aside.

Mix the soy flour, wheat gluten, baking powder, and salt together in a large basin using a whisk. Using your hands, stir in 3 tablespoons of olive oil and the warm yeast water. Add water gradually, one tablespoon at a time, until the dough is workable. Transfer to a bowl that has been greased and cover with plastic wrap. Put in a warm place and let it an hour to double in size. Pinch off the plastic wrap, flatten, reshape, and place onto the pizza pan. Prepare the topping while the dough is rising.

Turn the oven on to 450°F.

Regarding the garnish: Simmer one tablespoon of olive oil over medium heat in a skillet. Add the minced garlic to the pan and heat for 30 seconds. Next, add the chopped broccoli and cook for an additional two minutes. After removing from the heat, whisk in the ricotta cheese. After spreading the mixture over the crust, leaving a 1/2-inch border, sprinkle the Parmesan and mozzarella cheeses on top. Add oregano and the last tablespoon of oil on top. Bake for 20 to 22 minutes, or until well browned and puffed.

Keto Salmon and Green Bean Salad Recipe

Net Carbs	Prep Time	Cook Time	Phase	SERVINGS	Protein	Fat	Fiber	Calories
6.9g	15 Min	0 Min	Phase 1	4	20.7g	23.7g	4.6g	336.9cal

INGREDIENTS

1 fluid ounce Fresh Lemon Juice

2 teaspoons Dijon Mustard

1/3 cup Extra Virgin Olive Oil

3 cups Green Snap Beans

8 Cherry Tomatoes

2 tablespoons chopped Shallots

1 each Black Olives

4 tablespoons Basil

1/4 cup Parsley

1/8 teaspoon Salt

1/8 teaspoon Black Pepper

12 ounces Canned Salmon

6 cups Spring Mix Salad

3 ounces Roasted Bell Peppers

DIRECTIONS

Whisk together the mustard and lemon juice in a large bowl. Slowly pour in a tiny stream of olive oil and whisk continuously until smooth.

After steaming until perfectly soft, remove from heat and cut into 1-inch pieces. Dice the shallot finely, chop the parsley and basil, and cut the tomatoes in half.

Toss to coat all of the veggies and herbs in the dressing dish. Add salt and freshly ground black pepper to taste when seasoning.

Place fish in bowl after draining. To coat, gently toss.

Place greens on platters for serving. Add the salmon and green bean mixture over top. Add strips of roasted red pepper as a garnish.

Italian Chopped Salad Recipe

Net Carbs	Prep Time	Cook Time	Phase	SERVINGS	Protein	Fat	Fiber	Calories
8.2g	20 Min	0 Min	Phase 1	2	29.6g	28.4g	4.6g	420.4cal

INGREDIENTS

2 tablespoons Red Wine Vinegar

1 tablespoon Basil, fresh, chopped

1 tablespoon Parmesan Cheese, grated

1 teaspoon Dijon Mustard

1 tablespoon Olive Oil

1/2 cup Snap Peas, in pod, fresh, chopped

1 cup Cucumber, raw, sliced

10 each Cherry or Grape Tomato

2 ounces Mozzarella Cheese, fresh balls

1/2 package (4 oz) Hard Salami

4 ounces Chicken Roasted, dark and light meat

4 cups Romaine, raw, shredded

1 cup Baby Spinach

DIRECTIONS

Whisk the mustard with the vinegar, Parmesan, and chopped basil. Whisk the oil into the vinaigrette gradually. Put aside.

Chop the cooked chicken, salami, cucumber, tomatoes, mozzarella cheese, and peas into bite-sized pieces to prepare the veggies.

Combine the spinach and romaine lettuce with the dressing. Add the cheese, meats, and chopped veggies on top. Serve right away.

Chicken and Cheese Quesadillas Recipe

Net Carbs	Prep Time	Cook Time	Phase	SERVI NGS	Protein	Fat	Fiber	Calories
7.2g	5 Min	5 Min	Phase 2	4	34g	27.6g	8.3g	418.5cal

INGREDIENTS

1 cup shredded Monterey Jack Cheese
8 tortillas Low Carb Tortillas
8 ounces boneless, cooked Chicken Breast
2 ounces Roasted Bell Peppers
Three medium-sized (4-5/8-inch) spring onions
4 sprigs Cilantro
3 tablespoons Unsalted Butter Stick

DIRECTIONS

Partition and distribute half of the cheese among four tortillas, maintaining a 1/2-inch margin all around. Chop the scallions, roasted peppers, and chicken. Divide in half evenly, then lay on top of the cheese. Add the remaining cheese and cilantro and sprinkle. Take a tortilla and cover each.

For two minutes, preheat two large nonstick skillets over medium-high heat. Put a single slice of butter in each pan and warm it through. After placing one quesadilla in each pan, cook it for two to three minutes on each side, gently flipping it with a broad spatula. Continue with the remaining quesadillas and butter.

Make eight wedges out of each tortilla. Garnish with sour cream, salsa, tiny bell pepper, and jalapeño, if you'd like (but keep in mind that this will add more carbohydrates).

Turkey Tacos Recipe

Net Carbs	Prep Time	Cook Time	Phase	SERVINGS	Protein	Fat	Fiber	Calories
7.5g	10 Min	10 Min	Phase 2	4	39.5g	17.7g	4.8g	356.7cal

INGREDIENTS

2 tablespoons Light Olive Oil

16 oz, boneless, cooked, skinlesses Turkey Cutlet

1 tablespoon Original Taco Seasoning Mix

1/3 cup Sour Cream (Cultured)

1/4 cup chopped Red Onions

1 ounce Cilantro (Coriander)

4 tortillas Low Carb Tortillas

1/2 medium (approx 2-3/4" long, 2-1/2" diameter) Green Sweet Pepper

2 ounces Salsa

DIRECTIONS

In a large pan, heat 1 tablespoon (3 tablespoons) oil over medium-high heat. Taco seasoning should be added to the turkey cutlets before they are cooked through, which should take two minutes on each side. After moving the turkey to a chopping board, cut it into strips.

To the pan, add the sour cream, onion, and cilantro. Simmer for 3 minutes or until mixture is well cooked and onions are starting to soften.

Take the turkey strips back to the skillet with any liquids that have collected, mix to coat, and turn off the heat.

Heat 1 teaspoon oil in a medium pan over high heat until it's extremely hot before assembling each taco. Add tortilla and cook till light golden brown, one minute on each side. Eliminate and pour away surplus oil onto paper towels. Top with 1/4 of the pepper strips and 1 tablespoon of salsa after placing 1/4 of the contents on one side of the tortilla and folding it over. Use the leftover tortillas to repeat the whole procedure.

Keto Summer Chicken Salad Recipe

Net Carbs	Prep Time	Cook Time	Phase	SERVINGS	Protein	Fat	Fiber	Calories
4.6g	10 Min	0 Min	Phase 2	4	37.4g	23.9g	2.6g	389.4cal

INGREDIENTS

1 tablespoon Peanut Oil
2 teaspoons Sucralose Based Sweetener (Sugar Substitute)
1 1/2 teaspoons Salt
1/2 teaspoon Black Pepper
16 ounces boneless, cooked Chicken Breast
1 medium Carrot
16 tsp sugar-and sodium-free rice vinegar
4 cups shredded Chinese Cabbage (Bok-Choy, Pak-Choi)
1/4 cup Cilantro (Coriander)
1/4 cup Dry Roasted Unsalted Peanuts
2 tablespoons Toasted Sesame Oil
4 large Scallions or Spring Onions

DIRECTIONS

Note that cooked chicken breast is used in this recipe. A roasted chicken is available at the grocery shop.

Combine the oils, vinegar, sugar substitute, salt, and pepper in a big basin.

Add the peanuts, carrot, green onion, cilantro, bok choy, and chicken. Gently toss to mix.

Keto Beef Burger with Feta and Tomato Recipe

Net Carbs	Prep Time	Cook Time	Phase	SERVINGS	Protein	Fat	Fiber	Calories
1.2g	10 Min	12 Min	Phase 1	4	21.2g	24.7g	0.5g	318.7cal

INGREDIENTS

1 pound Ground Beef (80% Lean / 20% Fat)
1 large Scallions or Spring Onion
1/2 cup Baby Spinach
1/4 cup, chopped or sliced Red Tomatoes
1/4 cup, crumbled Feta Cheese
1/2 teaspoon Dill weed, dried
1/2 teaspoon Salt
1/2 teaspoon Black Pepper

DIRECTIONS

Add the ground beef, scallion, spinach, tomato, feta, salt, pepper, and 1.5 tsp fresh or 1/2 tsp dried dill. Shape into four patties.

For medium doneness, grill or pan-fry for six minutes on each side over medium-high heat.

Tofu Sautéed with Green Pepper, Scallions and Tamari Recipe

Net Carbs	Prep Time	Cook Time	Phase	SERVI NG	Protein	Fat	Fiber	Calories
9.3g	5 Min	10 Min	Phase 2	1	11.7g	16.8g	3.3g	243cal

INGREDIENTS

1 tablespoon Extra Virgin Olive Oil
4 ounces Firm Silken Tofu
3/4 cup chopped Green Sweet Pepper
1/2 cup chopped Scallions or Spring Onions
1 tablespoon Tamari Soybean Sauce

DIRECTIONS

Oil should be heated over medium-high heat in a nonstick skillet. Add the tofu and cook for five minutes, stirring occasionally, until golden brown.

Cook the green peppers and scallions for 3 to 4 minutes, or until the veggies are soft.

In the last minute of cooking, add tamari for seasoning. Serve right away.

Lettuce-Wrapped Swiss Cheeseburger with Tomato and Hummus Recipe

Net Carbs	Prep Time	Cook Time	Phase	SERVING	Protein	Fat	Fiber	Calories
8.7g	5 Min	10 Min	Phase 2	1	42.2g	47.3g	2.3g	647.7cal

INGREDIENTS

5 ounces Ground Beef (80% Lean / 20% Fat)
2 slice (1 ounce) Swiss Cheese
1 small whole (2-2/5" diameter) Red Tomato
2 tablespoons Organic Hummus Classic
3 leaves Butterhead Lettuce (Includes Boston and Bibb Types)

DIRECTIONS

Burger patties should be seasoned with salt and freshly ground black pepper. Burger should be cooked to desired doneness, approximately 5 minutes on each side.

For the last few minutes of cooking, cover with melted Swiss cheese.

Add hummus and tomato on top.

Encased with lettuce leaves.

Curried Fish and Red Peppers Over Broccoli Recipe

Net Carbs	Prep Time	Cook Time	Phase	SERVINGS	Protein	Fat	Fiber	Calories
8.1g	10 Min	15 Min	Phase 2	6	43.3g	17.5g	0.9g	354.3cal

INGREDIENTS

32 ounces Tilapia

6 cup flowerets Broccoli Flower Clusters

1 1/2 cups Coconut Cream, canned

1/2 tablespoon Roasted Red Chili Paste

2 teaspoons Ginger

1 1/2 tablespoons Fish Sauce

3 teaspoons Sucralose Based Sweetener (Sugar Substitute)

3 cups sliced Red Sweet Pepper

1/2 fluid ounce Fresh Lime Juice

DIRECTIONS

Season fish with a little amount of salt and freshly ground black pepper. Put aside.

Get a medium pot filled with water that has a steamer basket ready to boil. After the water reaches a boil, steam the broccoli for five to ten minutes, or until it is crisp-tender. As the broccoli steams, have the fish and sauce ready.

Add the coconut milk, chili paste, chopped ginger, lime juice, fish sauce, granulated sugar replacement, and bell peppers to a large sauté pan set over medium-high heat. After mixing the sauce ingredients and bringing it to a boil, add the fish. Fish should be cooked by basting it every two to three minutes with the sauce until the flesh is opaque and flake readily. After removing the fish to a platter, reduce the sauce over medium heat until it slightly thickens. Rewarm the fish in the pan for two to three minutes, squeeze in the lime juice, and serve right away with the broccoli.

Keto Baked Tofu with Cajun Rub Recipe

Net Carbs	Prep Time	Cook Time	Phase	SERVING	Protein	Fat	Fiber	Calories
5.3g	5 Min	30 Min	Phase 1	1	12.4g	9.6g	1.7g	160cal

INGREDIENTS

1 serving Keto Cajun Rub
6 ounces Firm Silken Tofu
1 teaspoon Extra Virgin Olive Oil

DIRECTIONS

To create Cajun Rub, follow the Atkins recipe; you'll need 1 tbsp.

Heat the oven to 375°.

Using a paper towel, drain and pat the tofu dry. Slice into strips that are 1/4 inch wide. If desired, rub oil and spice into the tofu and let it marinade for 30 minutes. Alternatively, season the tofu and cook it right away.

On a flat pan that has been oiled, bake for 15 minutes, then flip and continue baking for another 15 minutes, or until golden brown and somewhat crispy.

Wild Salmon Vera Cruz with Grilled Asparagus and Watercress Recipe

Net Carbs	Prep Time	Cook Time	Phase	SERVINGS	Protein	Fat	Fiber	Calories
10.5g	20 Min	10 Min	Phase 2	4	27.1g	59.2g	7.9g	732.8cal

INGREDIENTS

12 spear, medium (5-1/4" to 7" long) Asparagus

7 tablespoons Extra Virgin Olive Oil

1 teaspoon Salt

1 teaspoon Black Pepper

1 pound Wild Atlantic Salmon

1/2 cup chopped Sweet Red Peppers

10 cloves Garlic

1/2 cup chopped Onions

3 medium whole (2-3/5" diameter) Tomatoes

8 fluid ounces Sauvignon Blanc Wine

20 10 smalls Green Olives

2 tablespoons Butter

2 cups chopped Watercress

DIRECTIONS

Warm up the broiler or grill.

Add salt, pepper, and three tablespoons of virgin olive oil to the asparagus stalks and toss. Rolling occasionally, grill for 3–4 minutes, or until just tender. Place aside and maintain warmth.

Rinse and spin-dry the watercress in the meantime. Put aside.

In a large skillet or sauté pan, heat 3 tablespoons of the olive oil over medium-high heat.

Season the salmon with a pinch of salt and pepper. Put it in the skillet, flesh side down, and cook for two to three minutes, or until it becomes brown. Turn the salmon over.

Simmer the bell peppers, onions, diced tomatoes, garlic, and wine in a skillet with thinly sliced garlic. Cook the salmon, uncovered, for 4–5 minutes, or until it is medium rare.

Check the spices and add additional salt and pepper to taste. Add the olives and butter, stirring the butter frequently until it is absorbed.

Add a tablespoon of extra virgin olive oil and salt to the watercress.

Arrange three asparagus spears on each dish for serving. Evenly distribute a quarter of the sauce and a slice of salmon on top. Top each dish with a quarter of the watercress.

Keto Tequila Chicken Recipe

Net Carbs	Prep Time	Cook Time	Phase	SERVINGS	Protein	Fat	Fiber	Calories
1.5g	10 Min	15 Min	Phase 1	4	36.2g	48.6g	0.4g	613.3cal

INGREDIENTS

1/2 cup Canola Oil

1/4 cup Cilantro (Coriander)

1 1/2 fluid ounce (no ice) Tequila

1 1/2 tablespoons Cumin

3 teaspoons Garlic

1 teaspoon Salt

1/2 teaspoon Black Pepper

1/8 teaspoon Red or Cayenne Pepper

32 ounces uncooked (yield after cooking, without bone). Feline Breast

1/4 cup Unsalted Butter Stick

DIRECTIONS

Preheat the oven to 400°F.

Mix the oil, garlic, cumin, tequila, cilantro, salt, pepper, and cayenne in a big bowl. Toss in the chicken to coat.

Chicken should be moved to a baking sheet. Bake the biggest piece for 12 to 14 minutes, or until it is cooked through.

Take the breasts out of the oven, then place a tiny dollop of melted butter on top of each one.

Grilled Chicken over Baby Spinach, Tomato and Avocado Salad Recipe

Net Carbs	Prep Time	Cook Time	Phase	SERVI NG	Protein	Fat	Fiber	Calories
6g	5 Min	10 Min	Phase 1	1	57g	35.2g	10.8g	607.2cal

INGREDIENTS

1 serving Keto Sweet Mustard Dressing
6 ounces Chicken Breast Filet, skinless
2 cups Baby Spinach
1/2 large whole (3" diameter) Red Tomatoes
Half a fruit (no seeds and skin) that is a California avocado

DIRECTIONS

Make the Sweet Mustard Dressing according to the Atkins instructions; two teaspoons are required. Make sure the dressing you choose has less than 2g NC per serving (2 tbsp) if you want a different flavor.

Season the chicken with salt and freshly ground black pepper after preheating the grill.

Cook over medium heat until the center is no longer pink and the juices flow clear.

Mix the avocado, tomato, and baby spinach with the dressing. Add some cooked chicken on top, then serve right away.

Double Mushroom Soup Recipe

Net Carbs	Prep Time	Cook Time	Phase	SERVINGS	Protein	Fat	Fiber	Calories
5.4g	35 Min	45 Min	Phase 2	6	12.3g	16g	1.2g	217.7cal

INGREDIENTS

5 pieces Dried Porcini Mushrooms

Four cans (10.75 ounces), cooked according to the recipe Consomme, Bouillon, or Chicken Broth

3 tablespoons Unsalted Butter Stick

1 small Onion

12 ounces Mushroom Pieces and Stems

3 teaspoons Garlic

3 tablespoons Atkins Flour mix

1 teaspoon Thyme

1/4 teaspoon Nutmeg (Ground)

1/2 cup Heavy Cream

DIRECTIONS

Pour 14 1/2 ounces of chicken broth over the porcinis in a bowl and let stand for 30 minutes. Pour out the soaking liquid and reserve. Chop porcinis coarsely and reserve.

In a sauce saucepan over medium heat, melt the butter. Saute the button mushrooms and chopped onion for ten minutes. Simmer the minced garlic for a further thirty seconds. Stir in three tablespoons of Atkins Flour Mix; cook for two minutes. Stir in nutmeg, thyme, and the remaining 29 ounces of chicken broth, along with the saved porcini liquid gradually. After turning the heat up to high and bringing it to a boil, lower it to medium-low and simmer for five minutes. Add chopped porcinis to soup and boil until softened, about 10 more minutes.

Transfer half of the soup to a saucepan after blending it smooth in a food processor or blender. Simmer soup for three minutes after adding cream. To taste, add salt and pepper for seasoning.

Roasted Vegetable Soup Recipe

Net Carbs	Prep Time	Cook Time	Phase	SERVINGS	Protein	Fat	Fiber	Calories
6.7g	20 Min	75 Min	Phase 2	8	4.9g	17.3g	5.6g	212.3cal

INGREDIENTS

4 plum tomatoes Red Tomatoes

2 eggplant, unpeeled (approx 1-1/4 lb) Eggplant

4 cloves Garlic

3 tablespoons Light Olive Oil

1 1/4 teaspoons Marjoram (Dried)

2 14.5 ounces cans Chicken Broth, Bouillon or Consomme

1 cup Heavy Cream

3/4 teaspoon Salt

1/2 teaspoon Black Pepper

6 large Scallions or Spring Onions

DIRECTIONS

Preheat the oven to 400°F.

In a shallow roasting pan, arrange the tomatoes, eggplants, green onions, and garlic. Toss with marjoram and oil. Roast for 40 minutes, stirring regularly, or until veggies are soft and beginning to turn brown. After the eggplants have cooled down enough, remove the pulp and place it in a large saucepot. Include the other veggies.

Add broth and stir. Bring over high heat to a boil. Vegetables should be simmered for 35 minutes over low heat to become very tender. Nice.

Blend soup in batches using a blender. Put the soup back in the saucepot. Add cream, pepper, and salt, and stir. Warm up thoroughly.

Keto Smoky Tuna Tomato Recipe

Net Carbs	Prep Time	Cook Time	Phase	SERVINGS	Protein	Fat	Fiber	Calories
2.3g	10 Min	0 Min	Phase 1	2	26.8g	33.1g	1.1g	421.3cal

INGREDIENTS

1 medium whole (2-3/5" diameter) Red Tomato
6 ounces Tuna in Water (Canned)
1 tablespoon chopped Chives
6 tablespoons Real Mayonnaise
3 tablespoons Real Bacon Bits
1/2 fluid ounce Fresh Lemon Juice
1/2 each Chipotle en Adobo, whole
1/8 teaspoon Salt

DIRECTIONS

Halve the tomato and remove the seeds and pulp with a spoon. Sprinkle salt and pepper on top (optional) and drizzle with a little olive oil.

Dice the chipotle pepper finely and transfer to a small dish with the other ingredients (dry the tuna first, of course). After blending until well combined, spoon tuna mixture into tomato halves and serve.

Keto Baked Tofu with Latin Marinade Recipe

Net Carbs	Prep Time	Cook Time	Phase	SERVING	Protein	Fat	Fiber	Calories
5.6g	5 Min	30 Min	Phase 1	1	12g	25.6g	0.4g	299.1cal

INGREDIENTS

1 serving Keto Latin Marinade
6 ounces Firm Silken Tofu

DIRECTIONS

Using a paper towel, drain and pat the tofu dry. After cutting into 1/4-inch strips, marinate them.

Turn the oven on to 375° 3. If desired, marinate the tofu for at least thirty minutes.
On a flat pan that has been oiled, bake for 15 minutes, then flip and continue baking for another 15 minutes, or until golden brown and somewhat crispy. To use on a salad or to reheat for a warm meal, serve right away or keep in the refrigerator for up to three days.

Raspberry Parfait Recipe

Net Carbs	Prep Time	Cook Time	Phase	SERVINGS	Protein	Fat	Fiber	Calories
4.2g	5 Min	0 Min	Phase 2	2	5.6g	46.2g	2g	464.6cal

INGREDIENTS

1/2 cup Heavy Cream

4 ounces Mascarpone

2 individual packets Sucralose Based Sweetener (Sugar Substitute)

1/2 cup Raspberries

DIRECTIONS

Up until soft peaks form, beat 1/2 cup heavy cream.

Stir in 2 packets of sugar and 4 ounces of mascarpone. Beat just till smooth. If desired, taste and add extra sweetness.

Line two parfait glasses with the dairy mixture and top with half a cup of raspberries.

Please wait, Your Review is Very Important…

Dear Reader,

I hope this message finds you well. Thank you for choosing to read the Atkins Diet Book for Beginners 2024. Your feedback is incredibly valuable to me, and I would love to hear your thoughts on the book. Whether you've just started, are halfway through, or have finished reading, your perspective matters.

Your feedback is immensely appreciated and will help me enhance future works.

Thank you for taking the time to share your thoughts on the Atkins Diet Book for Beginners 2024. Your support means the world to me.

Happy reading!

Dr. Valerie Kennedy

Chapter 6: Snacks and Desserts

Keto Chocolate Caramel Pretzel Cookie Bars Recipe

Net Carbs	Prep Time	Cook Time	Phase	SERVINGS	Protein	Fat	Fiber	Calories
1.5g	85 Min	26 Min	Phase 2	12	2.7g	11.7g	3.1g	127.8cal

INGREDIENTS

6 tablespoons butter, unsalted

1/3 cup allulose, granulated Wholesome

1 teaspoon vanilla extract

1/4 teaspoon table salt

3/4 cup of very finely milled, gluten-free almond flour

2 tablespoons coconut flour, finely ground, organic

1/4 teaspoon xanthan gum

47 grams semisweet style chocolate baking chips, 45% cocoa, no sugar added

1 bar Atkins Chocolate Caramel Pretzel Snack Bar

DIRECTIONS

Preheat the oven to 325°F. Line a 7 ½ by 6 inch baking dish with baking parchment.

Melted butter, granulated allulose, vanilla extract, and salt should all be blended well in a medium-sized dish so that there are no sweetener clumps left. Mix in the xanthan gum, coconut flour, and almond flour until a thick dough develops and all of the flour is well combined. Evenly spread into the baking dish that has been prepared.

Bake for fifteen minutes, then turn and continue baking for ten more minutes, or until the tops are golden brown. In the last five minutes, keep a close eye to make sure it doesn't burn.

Take out of the oven, shut it off, then add the chocolate chips and return to the oven for another two minutes, or until the chips are shiny. After letting the cookie cool in the baking sheet for five minutes, cover it with an even coating of melted chocolate using an offset spatula or rubber scraper. Add sea salt flakes and coarsely diced Atkins Chocolate Caramel Pretzel bar on top. Allow it cool for an additional fifteen minutes in the pan, then take it out and allow it cool fully for an additional hour. Finally, cut into twelve equal pieces. A single piece equals one serving.

Keto Chocolate Pecan Shortbread Drops Recipe

Net Carbs	Prep Time	Cook Time	Phase	SERVINGS	Protein	Fat	Fiber	Calories
0.7g	20 Min	14 Min	Phase 2	50	1.2g	4.9g	0.5g	50.7cal

INGREDIENTS

16 tablespoons Unsalted Butter Stick

1/2 cup Sucralose Based Sweetener (Sugar Substitute)

1/2 teaspoon stevia sweetener

1 large Egg (Whole)

2 tablespoons Cream, heavy, liquid

1 teaspoon Vanilla Extract

3/4 cup(s) defatted soy flour (1 cup= 105g)

Three tsp straight phosphate, double-acting baking powder

3 tablespoons Cocoa Powder

1/2 cup chopped Pecan Nuts

DIRECTIONS

Turn the oven on to 325°F.

Using an electric mixer, beat butter, stevia, and sucralose on medium speed for about four minutes, or until light and fluffy. Reduce the speed to low and mix in the egg, cream, vanilla, and optional 1 tsp chocolate essence. After scraping down the sides of the bowl, stir in the soy flour, baking powder, cocoa powder, and pecans until just incorporated.

Spoon dough onto ungreased baking sheets in heaping teaspoonfuls. Cook for 12 to 14 minutes, or until the cookies are firm. Allow to cool for one minute on the sheets, then move to wire racks to finish cooling.

Vanilla Mousse with Rhubarb Sauce Recipe

Net Carbs	Prep Time	Cook Time	Phase	SERVINGS	Protein	Fat	Fiber	Calories
7.5g	15 Min	10 Min	Phase 2	2	7.3g	22.1g	1.9g	253.7cal

INGREDIENTS

2 stalks Rhubarb

1/4 cup Tap Water

1 tablespoon Sugar Free Strawberry Jam

1/2 cup Heavy Cream

4 ounces Greek Yogurt - Plain (Container)

3 teaspoons Sucralose Based Sweetener (Sugar Substitute)

DIRECTIONS

To make the rhubarb sauce, put the rhubarb, water, and strawberry jam in a small saucepan and cook it to a simmer over medium heat. Lower the heat to medium-low, cover, and simmer for approximately 10 minutes, stirring now and again, until the rhubarb takes on the consistency of sauce. Put aside to cool.

To make the vanilla mousse, whisk the cream, 4 ounces of yogurt, and sugar substitute in a mixing bowl on medium-high speed with an electric mixer until semi-firm peaks form. Set aside 1/4 cup mousse for the garnish.

To put together: Arrange two wineglasses or martini glasses. Evenly distribute 1/4 cup of mousse in the bottom of each glass using a spoon. Add 1 1/2 teaspoons of rhubarb sauce on top of each. Spoon the leftover mousse into each glass, then garnish with the remaining rhubarb. Evenly divide the 1/4 cup mousse that was set aside on top.

Walnut Blondies Recipe

Net Carbs	Prep Time	Cook Time	Phase	SERVINGS	Protein	Fat	Fiber	Calories
5.2g	20 Min	14 Min	Phase 3	12	8.7g	26.2g	2.1g	286.5cal

INGREDIENTS

1 cup chopped English Walnuts

1 cup Unsalted Butter Stick

1 cup Sucralose Based Sweetener (Sugar Substitute)

1 teaspoon Vanilla Extract

1 cup Whole Grain Soy Flour

1/2 cup 100% Stone Ground Whole Wheat Pastry Flour

3 large Eggs (Whole)

1 ounce Vital Wheat Gluten

1 1/2 teaspoons Baking Powder (Straight Phosphate, Double Acting)

1/2 teaspoon Cinnamon

2 servings Unsweetened Baking Chocolate Squares

DIRECTIONS

Preheat the oven to 325°F. On a sheet pan, toast the walnuts for 8 to 10 minutes. Once cooled, finely chop them. Put aside.

Aluminum foil should reach 2 inches over both short edges of a 13 by 9-inch baking pan. Oil the foil and keep it aside.

In a large bowl, whisk together butter, sugar substitute, eggs, and vanilla extract. incorporate the flours, baking powder, gluten, and cinnamon in a separate dish, then thoroughly incorporate them into the butter mixture. Add walnuts and stir. Evenly spread into the pan that has been prepared. Bake for 12 to 14 minutes, or until puffed and set and a toothpick inserted in the middle comes out clean (top will not brown).

Leave the pan on a wire rack to cool completely. Over the whole surface of the brownies, drizzle chocolate in thin lines. Let stand for approximately an hour or until set. (Up to this stage, the recipe may be made, wrapped with cutting into 12 pieces, serve.

plastic wrap, and left overnight at room temperature.)

Blondies should be taken out of the pan and placed on a work surface with both ends of the foil firmly gripped. After

Strawberries with French Cream Recipe

Net Carbs	Prep Time	Cook Time	Phase	SERVINGS	Protein	Fat	Fiber	Calories
6.4g	10 Min	0 Min	Phase 2	4	1.5g	13.1g	1.7g	150.4cal

INGREDIENTS

1/2 cup Heavy Cream

1 tablespoon Sucralose Based Sweetener (Sugar Substitute)

3 tablespoons Sour Cream (Cultured)

12 ounces fresh strawberries

DIRECTIONS

Beat cream and sugar on high speed for approximately 4 minutes, or until soft peaks form.

Mix in sour cream well by beating. Accompany with berries.

Raspberry Parfait Recipe

Net Carbs	Prep Time	Cook Time	Phase	SERVINGS	Protein	Fat	Fiber	Calories
4.2g	5 Min	0 Min	Phase 2	2	5.6g	46.2g	2g	464.6cal

INGREDIENTS

1/2 cup Heavy Cream

4 ounces Mascarpone

2 individual packets Sucralose Based Sweetener (Sugar Substitute)

1/2 cup Raspberries

DIRECTIONS

Up until soft peaks form, beat 1/2 cup heavy cream.

Stir in 2 packets of sugar and 4 ounces of mascarpone. Beat just till smooth. If desired, taste and add extra sweetness.

Line two parfait glasses with the dairy mixture and top with half a cup of raspberries.

Low Carb Irish Coffee Recipe

Net Carbs	Prep Time	Cook Time	Phase	SERVINGS	Protein	Fat	Fiber	Calories
1g	5 Min	10 Min	Phase 2	6	0.6g	7.3g	0g	176cal

INGREDIENTS

36 fluid ounces Decaffeinated Coffee
9 fluid ounce (no ice) Whiskey
3 teaspoons Sucralose Based Sweetener (Sugar Substitute)
1/2 cup Heavy Cream

DIRECTIONS

Make 4 ½ cups (36 fl oz) of coffee and keep it warm.

Whiskey (9 fl oz, or 1 cup plus 2 teaspoons) should be warmed in a small saucepan over medium-low heat; do not boil. Blend warm whiskey and sugar substitute into freshly made coffee.

Lightly whip heavy cream to soft peaks in the small bowl of an electric mixer set on medium speed.

Approximately 7 ½ fluid ounces, or slightly less than 1 cup each serving, of the coffee mixture should be divided among 6 cups. Place a dollop of whipped cream (approximately 2 tablespoons per serving) on top of each cup.

Atkins Pie Crust Recipe

Net Carbs	Prep Time	Cook Time	Phase	SERVINGS	Protein	Fat	Fiber	Calories
3.6g	65 Min	16 Min	Phase 3	8	8.6g	13.2g	1.3g	168.2cal

INGREDIENTS

1/3 cup 100% Stone Ground Whole Wheat Pastry Flour
1/3 cup Whole Grain Soy Flour
2 ounces Vital Wheat Gluten
3 tablespoons Plain Wheat Germ
1/2 teaspoon Salt
1/2 cup Unsalted Butter Stick
1 tablespoon Tap Water

DIRECTIONS

Pulse flours, butter, wheat germ, gluten, and salt in a food processor until the mixture resembles coarse meal. Water should be added gradually while pulsing the dough until it starts to come together. Transfer to a plastic wrap sheet, roll into a ball, and wrap in plastic. Press into a 7-inch round and freeze for fifteen minutes.

Roll out the dough to a 12-inch circle between two pieces of plastic wrap; if necessary, dust each side with 1/2 teaspoon of wheat gluten flour to make rolling easier. Take off the top plastic sheet and turn the mixture over into a 9-inch pie pan. Press the dough into the center of the plate's sides and bottom. Take off the plastic, roll the edges under, and add ornamental crimps. For fifteen minutes, let it cool in the freezer.

Prepare the unbaked crust according to the recipe's instructions. Alternately, preheat the oven to 400° F for a prebaked crust. Using a fork, prick the pie shell's edges and bottom. Pie weights or dry beans may be used to partially fill a lined pie shell. Then, flip the foil over to cover the pastry border. Bake for sixteen minutes.

After removing the weights and foil, bake for a further 4 to 6 minutes, or until brown. Loosely cover with foil. Before using, let cool on a rack for 20 minutes. Yields eight servings.

Double Chocolate Pecan Ice Cream Recipe

Net Carbs	Prep Time	Cook Time	Phase	SERVINGS	Protein	Fat	Fiber	Calories
7.6g	300 Min	18 Min	Phase 2	8	7.1g	44.3g	5.3g	446.9cal

INGREDIENTS

1 cup chopped Pecans

1 teaspoon Gelatin Powder

1 cup Tap Water

6 large Egg Yolks

3/4 cup Sucralose Based Sweetener (Sugar Substitute)

2 1/2 cups Heavy Cream

2/3 cup Cocoa Powder (Unsweetened)

1/2 teaspoon Salt

1 1/2 teaspoons Vanilla Extract

4 tablespoons Lily's Sugar Free Chocolate Chips

DIRECTIONS

Set the oven to 350°F.

After 8 minutes of toasting, take out and let cool, then cut and save the pecans. Pour the gelatin into a heavy-bottomed saucepan of water. Let stand for approximately five minutes, or until softened.

Whisk together the yolks and sugar substitute in a medium-sized bowl. To the gelatin mixture, add the cream and cocoa powder. Cook over medium-low heat, stirring regularly, until the cocoa is dissolved and the liquid starts to boil.

While continuously whisking, slowly add half of the gelatin mixture into the yolk mixture. Refill the pot with the mixture. We call this procedure tempering. Cook for approximately 4 minutes, stirring continuously, or until mixture is thick enough to coat the back of a spoon. Take off the heat.

Add the chocolate, vanilla, and salt extracts and stir. Mixture should be chilled for four hours. Fill the ice cream machine with ice cream. Follow the manufacturer's instructions for processing. When the ice cream is almost done, add the chocolate and pecans.

Keto Coconut Thumbprints Recipe

Net Carbs	Prep Time	Cook Time	Phase	SERVINGS	Protein	Fat	Fiber	Calories
0.9g	20 Min	8 Min	Phase 2	36	1.3g	5.7g	0.7g	60cal

INGREDIENTS

2/3 cup, shelled (32 kernels) Brazil Nuts

1/2 cup Coconut, shredded, unsweetened

1/2 cup Whole Grain Soy Flour

Two and a half teaspoons of sucrose-based sweetener (sugar alternative)

1/2 cup Unsalted Butter Stick

1 large Egg (Whole)

1 large Egg Yolk

1 teaspoon Coconut Extract

3 tablespoons Sugar Free Seedless Blackberry Jam

DIRECTIONS

Turn the oven on to 375°F.

Pulse 1/2 cup coconut and nuts in a food processor for about one minute, or until finely ground. Pulse to blend in the sugar replacement and soy flour.

When the mixture resembles a coarse grain, add the butter and pulse for a further 30 seconds. Add the egg, yolk, and extract, and pulse for one minute, or until the dough barely comes together.

Scrape dough into basin; cover and refrigerate until somewhat hard, at least 3 hours. Create 36 spheres out of the dough, then place them on an ungreased baking sheet. Make a depression in the middle of each ball, like a doughnut, by dipping your thumb into warm water (don't push all the way through).

Put a tsp of jam in each depression. Bake for approximately 6 minutes, or until brown. Allow to cool for one minute on the baking sheet, then move to wire racks to finish cooling.

Keto Chocolate Ganache Macarons Recipe

Net Carbs	Prep Time	Cook Time	Phase	SERVINGS	Protein	Fat	Fiber	Calories
1.1g	15 Min	40 Min	Phase 1	20	1.8g	4g	2.6g	49.8cal

INGREDIENTS

3 large Egg Whites
1 teaspoon Fresh Lemon Juice
2 tablespoons Xylitol
3/4 cup Almond Meal Flour
6 tablespoons Lily's Sugar Free Chocolate Chips
2 tablespoons Heavy Cream

DIRECTIONS

Turn the oven on to 250°F. Line a baking sheet with parchment paper or a silicon baking mat. It might be useful to draw 1-inch circles on the parchment's reverse side. Put aside.

The egg whites, lemon juice, a small sprinkle of salt, and one tablespoon, or three tsp, of xylitol should be whipped using a stand mixer fitted with the whip attachment until firm peaks form.

Almond flour and the last tablespoon of xylitol should be sifted together. To properly combine, add to the egg whites and fold in gently. Pipe 1-inch circles onto the baking sheet using a piping bag or just cutting the end of a big zipped plastic bag filled with meringue. If tips remain, tap the tops with a finger that's somewhat damp. For 35 to 45 minutes, bake. Reduce the oven temperature by 25 degrees and continue baking if they start to brown. Take out of the oven and let cool. After cooling, remove with a spatula and place on a new parchment paper sheet.

Produce Filling: heat chocolate for 30 seconds at a time. Using a handheld blender, add the heavy cream and whisk until thickened. Pipe chocolate into one macaron's flat side using a tiny piping bag, then top with another macaron so that they are sandwiched together on the flat side. If preferred, add a little pinch of cocoa powder as a garnish. 1 macaron equals 1 portion.

Strawberry Granita Recipe

Net Carbs	Prep Time	Cook Time	Phase	SERVINGS	Protein	Fat	Fiber	Calories
7.2g	120 Min	0 Min	Phase 2	6	0.5g	0.2g	1.5g	34.8cal

INGREDIENTS

16 ounces Strawberries
1 cup Tap Water
3/4 cup Sucralose Based Sweetener (Sugar Substitute)
1 tablespoon Fresh Lemon Juice

DIRECTIONS

Puree the strawberries in a food processor that has a steel blade attached. Add the lemon juice, water, and sugar substitute. To blend, pulse.

Fill a 9 by 13-inch baking pan with ingredients. Put it in the freezer. Set aside 30 minutes to freeze. Use a fork to stir. For a further one and a half to two hours, freeze the mixture, scraping it down with a fork every thirty minutes to break up any big pieces.

If preferred, top with sprigs of mint and serve in dessert plates.

Coconut Pie Recipe

Net Carbs	Prep Time	Cook Time	Phase	SERVINGS	Protein	Fat	Fiber	Calories
9.3g	30 Min	20 Min	Phase 2	8	12.2g	41.3g	3.8g	473.4cal

INGREDIENTS

1 1/2 cups almond meal, super fine, with skin

1 3/4 cups Coconut, shredded, unsweetened

3/4 cup Sucralose Based Sweetener (Sugar Substitute)

1 large Egg White

1 tablespoon coconut oil

1 1/4 cups canned coconut cream

1/2 cup Heavy Cream

6 large Eggs (Whole)

1 large Egg Yolk

1 teaspoon Vanilla Extract

1 teaspoon Coconut Extract

1/4 teaspoon Salt

DIRECTIONS

For crust

Preheat the oven to 350°F. Grease a 9-inch pie pan very lightly.

Combine almond meal, melted coconut oil, egg white, 1/4 cup sugar replacement, and one cup shredded coconut. Add one to two tablespoons of water, a few drops at a time, if the mixture is too dry to keep together, until it retains its form when pressed together.

Form a crust by pressing equally onto the bottom and up the edges of the prepared pie dish. For fifteen minutes, bake until gently browned. Take out of oven and put aside. Raise the oven's setting to 450°F.

For completing

In a medium saucepan, simmer the coconut milk and cream over medium heat, stirring often, until little bubbles start to form around the pan's edges or the temperature reaches 180–185°. Then, remove from the heat and allow the mixture to cool somewhat.

Beat the eggs and egg yolk in a large bowl using a wire whisk or an electric mixer set on medium speed until frothy. Add the salt, vanilla, and coconut extract, and beat in 1/2 cup sugar replacement. Beat in the heated coconut milk mixture gradually.

Stir carefully and fold in all but 2 tablespoons of the remaining 3/4 cup of coconut shreds. After adding the filling to the prepared crust, top with the last two tablespoons of shredded coconut. Bake at 450°F for 5 minutes. Bake for a further 15 minutes at 350°F. Keep an eye on the crust for the last ten minutes, and if necessary, wrap a piece of foil over the edge to keep it from burning. When the middle of the pie is easily cut with a knife and the internal temperature hits 160°, the pie is done. Place in the refrigerator to cool entirely after allowing it to cool to room temperature on a wire rack. Yields eight servings.

Cherry Hazelnut Biscotti Recipe

Net Carbs	Prep Time	Cook Time	Phase	SERVINGS	Protein	Fat	Fiber	Calories
4.3g	45 Min	73 Min	Phase 2	16	4.2g	13.9g	2.1g	157.9cal

INGREDIENTS

1 1/2 cups hazelnuts, chopped

1 cup almond flour, super finely ground, gluten free

1/3 cup sucralose artificial sweetener, granular

2 tablespoons coconut flour, finely ground, organic

1/2 teaspoon cinnamon, ground

1/4 teaspoon table salt

2 lrgs raw egg

3 tablespoons butter, unsalted

2 tablespoons sour cream

1/4 cup dried cherries, organic, unsweetened

DIRECTIONS

Preheat the oven to 350°F. A baking sheet should be lined with parchment paper.

One cup of the hazelnuts should be cut finely; set aside half a cup for coarsely chopped hazelnuts. Put in a big bowl and mix in the coconut flour, ground cinnamon, almond flour, granulated sugar, and salt. Stir well after adding the sour cream, eggs, and melted butter. The dough will be dense and sticky. Stir in the remaining ½ cup of coarsely chopped hazelnuts and chopped cherries.

Shape the dough into an 8-inch-long, 4-inch-wide, and ¾-inch-high log on the prepared baking sheet. Bake for 25 to 30 minutes, or until well-done. Place on a wire rack and let cool for half an hour.

Lower the oven's setting to 300°F. Using a serrated knife, carefully cut the logs crosswise into 16 and a half-inch broad slices. Place slices on the baking pan, then bake for nine minutes. After 9 to 15 minutes, flip and continue cooking until the bottoms are well browned. For at least another half hour, let the biscotti cool gently and crisp by inserting a wooden spoon inside the door and turning the oven off. A single biscotti slice represents a dish.

Chocolate Yule Log Recipe

Net Carbs	Prep Time	Cook Time	Phase	SERVINGS	Protein	Fat	Fiber	Calories
5.7g	20 Min	12 Min	Phase 2	10	8.2g	28.9g	1.8g	307.9cal

INGREDIENTS

1 1/3 cups Sucralose Based Sweetener (Sugar Substitute)
5 tablespoons Cocoa Powder (Unsweetened)
9 large Eggs (Whole)
2 tablespoons Whole Grain Soy Flour
1/4 teaspoon Salt
1 1/3 cups Heavy Cream
2 ounces Unsweetened Baking Chocolate Squares
8 tablespoons Unsalted Butter Stick
1/4 teaspoon Vanilla Extract

DIRECTIONS

Turn the oven on to 375°F. Grease a jelly roll pan with cooking spray; cover with parchment paper, leaving a 2-inch edge; reapply oil spray. Put aside.

Combine 1 cup sugar replacement, 4 tablespoons cocoa powder, and soy flour in a big bowl.

Egg yolks should be beaten with an electric mixer on high speed for three minutes or until they are light yellow and frothy in another big basin. Reduce the speed to low and stir in the cocoa mixture very gently, just until incorporated.

Use an electric mixer to whip the egg whites and salt in a separate bowl on high speed for about three minutes, or until firm peaks form. Just incorporate 1/3 of the whites with the yolk mixture by folding them in. Blend in the leftover egg whites. Pour batter into prepared pan evenly. Bake for 15 minutes, or until the cake comes away from the pan's sides and bounces back when gently touched. Allow the cake to cool in the pan on a wire rack for half an hour or more.

Prepare the icing and filling while the cake cools. In a medium bowl, whisk together 1 cup cream and 1/2 tablespoon sugar substitute until firm peaks form, being careful not to overbeat.

In a large dish, gently stir together 1/3 cup cream and melted chocolate to make the frosting. Beat in butter, 5 tablespoons sugar replacement, 1 tablespoon cocoa powder, and vanilla with an electric mixer set at medium speed. Beat for approximately 4

minutes, or until fluffy and smooth. Store in the refrigerator until needed.

After the cake cools, remove it from the pan using the paper below. Put it on the counter. Cover cake with filling, leaving ½ inch border around edge. Roll the cake from the narrow end, assisting with the parchment. From each end, cut diagonal sections 1 inch long. After transferring the roll to a serving tray, create log stumps by placing sliced diagonal slices on each side. Put aside.

To put together: Apply a thick layer of icing to affix the stumps to the main log. Cover the whole log with icing, then use a fork to create a texture like bark.

Pear Tart Recipe

Net Carbs	Prep Time	Cook Time	Phase	SERVINGS	Protein	Fat	Fiber	Calories
13.3g	40 Min	30 Min	Phase 3	6	11.3g	32.5g	4.2g	403.7cal

INGREDIENTS

3/4 cup Whole Grain Soy Flour

9 tablespoons Sucralose Based Sweetener (Sugar Substitute)

4 tablespoons Unsalted Butter Stick

11 ounces Cream Cheese

1 tablespoon Sour Cream (Cultured)

2 small pear (approx 3 per lb) Pear

1 fluid ounce (no ice) Brandy

1/2 teaspoon Pure Almond Extract

1/2 teaspoon Ginger (Ground)

2 tablespoons Sugar Free Apricot Preserves

1 large Egg (Whole)

2 teaspoons Tap Water

1 ounce Almonds

DIRECTIONS

Turn the oven on to 350°F.

To make the crust, blend 2 tablespoons sugar substitute and flour in a food processor for approximately 10 seconds. Add butter and process for 30 seconds or until mixture resembles coarse grain.

Incorporate 3 ounces of cream cheese and sour cream, pulsing for an additional 30 seconds or until the dough begins to come together. Press the dough into an ungreased 10-tart pan, covering the bottom and the edges.

While making the filling, prick the dough with a fork approximately fifteen times and place it in the freezer.

To make the filling, combine the pear slices, 1/4 teaspoon of almond essence, brandy or Cognac, and ginger in a small bowl and mix until well distributed. Put aside.

Beat 1/3 cup sugar substitute and 8 ounces room-temperature cream cheese in a large bowl using an electric mixer set on high speed until the mixture is smooth and creamy, which should take approximately 3 minutes. After adding the egg and the remaining 1/4 teaspoon almond extract, beat for another minute or until smooth, scraping down the sides of the basin as needed.

Fill the cooled tart shell with the cream cheese mixture. Place pears in concentric rings that slightly overlap on top of the cream cheese mixture. Pour any remaining juice from the pears evenly over the tart.

Bake until the cheese mixture is barely set, about 30 minutes. Take out of the oven and let cool on a wire rack.

Melt jam in a pan over medium heat with water. Drizzle the heated tart with the glaze and top with almonds. Let the tart cool completely before slicing.

Bittersweet Chocolate Brownie Drops Recipe

Net Carbs	Prep Time	Cook Time	Phase	SERVINGS	Protein	Fat	Fiber	Calories
2.9g	15 Min	10 Min	Phase 3	12	2.6g	9.3g	1.1g	100cal

INGREDIENTS

2 tablespoons 100% Stone Ground Whole Wheat Pastry Flour
2 tablespoons Whole Grain Soy Flour
1/4 teaspoon Baking Powder (Straight Phosphate, Double Acting)
3 ounces Unsweetened Baking Chocolate Squares
6 tablespoons Heavy Cream
2 tablespoons Unsalted Butter Stick
2 large Eggs (Whole)
3/4 cup Sucralose Based Sweetener (Sugar Substitute)

DIRECTIONS

Turn the oven on to 375°F. Use aluminum foil or parchment paper to line a baking pan.

Mix the baking powder, soy flour, and two tablespoons of flour in a big basin.

Melt the chocolate, cream, and butter in a microwave-safe dish for one to two minutes, or until the butter is melted and the chocolate has softened. After two minutes, let stand and stir until smooth. This stage may also be completed on a cooktop.

Beat eggs and sugar substitute for three minutes on medium speed with an electric mixer, or until light and fluffy. Beat the somewhat warm chocolate mixture into the egg mixture gradually until well combined, which should take approximately a minute. Reduce the speed of your mixer to low and quickly mix in the flour mixture.

Drop dough onto the prepared sheet in gently rounded teaspoonfuls. Bake for 5–6 minutes, or until the top is slightly

soft but the center is set. Transfer to a
wire rack to cool completely.

Pumpkin Mousse Recipe

Net Carbs	Prep Time	Cook Time	Phase	SERVINGS	Protein	Fat	Fiber	Calories
5.7g	120 Min	10 Min	Phase 1	8	2.3g	16.7g	1.6g	184.4cal

INGREDIENTS

1 envelope Gelatin, unsweetened
1/4 cup Tap Water
2 teaspoons Pumpkin Pie Spice
15 ounces Pumpkin (Without Salt, Canned)
1 1/2 cups Heavy Cream
1/2 cup Sucralose Based Sweetener (Sugar Substitute)
2 teaspoons Vanilla Extract

DIRECTIONS

Pour cold water over the gelatin in a small bowl and let it rest for five minutes to soften. Meanwhile, toast the pumpkin pie spice in a small pan over medium heat for one to two minutes, turning regularly, until fragrant. Simmer for a further one to two minutes, stirring, over low heat until the gelatin has melted. Take off the heat and let it reach room temperature.

Put the puréed pumpkin in a big basin.

Using an electric mixer set to high speed in a separate large bowl, whip together the cream, sugar substitute, and vanilla until soft peaks form. Gradually fold in the chilled gelatin mixture using a rubber spatula.

Gently incorporate whipped cream mixture into pumpkin purée in three increments. Pour mousse into eight dessert goblets. Relax for two hours.

Frozen Chocolate Fudge Tart Recipe

Net Carbs	Prep Time	Cook Time	Phase	SERVINGS	Protein	Fat	Fiber	Calories
5.9g	210 Min	20 Min	Phase 2	12	6.8g	29.4g	4.4g	310.6cal

INGREDIENTS

1/2 serving Atkins Soy-Free Flour Mix

5 tablespoons Cocoa Powder (Unsweetened)

1/2 teaspoon Cinnamon

7 tablespoons Sucralose Based Sweetener (Sugar Substitute)

4 tablespoons Unsalted Butter Stick

3 ounces Cream Cheese

4 ounces Lily's Sugar Free Chocolate Chips

2 teaspoons Vanilla Extract

2 1/2 cups Heavy Cream

1 teaspoon dried Coffee (Instant Powder)

DIRECTIONS

Turn the oven on to 425°F. After cutting a circle of parchment paper to fit into the bottom of a 9-inch pie pan, oil the pie plate, then insert the parchment.

Regarding the crust: Pulse the 1/2 cup baking mix, 4 teaspoons cocoa powder, cinnamon, and 3 tablespoons sugar substitute in a food processor for about 10 seconds to blend. Add the cold, chopped butter and pulse for 30 seconds or until the mixture resembles coarse grain. Add the cream cheese and pulse for a further 30 seconds or until the mixture starts to come together.

Spoon dough into a 9-inch pie pan that has been prepped, pressing into an equal layer on the edges and bottom. Using a fork, prick the dough around fifteen times, then decoratively crimp the edges. Bake for ten minutes, or until set, with a light cover of aluminum foil on. Remove the lid and continue baking for an additional 8 to 10 minutes, until the color becomes light golden brown. Before filling, let the crust cool.

To make the filling, combine one teaspoon of vanilla essence with chocolate in a medium-sized dish. For approximately four minutes, over medium-high heat, cook one cup of cream and instant coffee until they are almost boiling. After pouring over the chocolate and waiting three minutes, stir to melt the chocolate. Fill pie shell, level top, and refrigerate for half an hour.

Beat the remaining cream, 4 tablespoons sugar substitute, 1 teaspoon vanilla extract, and 1 tablespoon cocoa powder in a medium bowl on high speed with an electric mixer until medium peaks form, approximately 4 minutes. Cover with a coating of chocolate and freeze for a minimum of 2.5 hours, or until solid. Ten minutes before serving, take out of the freezer.

Whole-Grain Tart Shell Recipe

Net Carbs	Prep Time	Cook Time	Phase	SERVINGS	Protein	Fat	Fiber	Calories
1.7g	30 Min	20 Min	Phase 3	10	9.1g	10g	0.2g	132cal

INGREDIENTS

1/2 cup 100% Stone Ground Whole Wheat Pastry Flour
4 ounces Vital Wheat Gluten
1 tablespoon Whole Grain Soy Flour
1/4 teaspoon Salt
1/2 cup Unsalted Butter Stick
1 large Egg Yolk
1/8 fluid ounce Tap Water

DIRECTIONS

Pulse the flours, butter, and salt in a food processor until the mixture resembles coarse meal. After adding the yolk and water, pulse the dough until it just begins to come together.

Place the dough onto a large plastic wrap sheet, shape it into a ball, and then cover it with another plastic wrap sheet. Press into a 7-inch round and freeze for ten minutes.

Roll out the dough between the plastic wrap to a 13-inch circle (sometimes remove the film and sprinkle each side with 1/2 tsp wheat gluten flour to make rolling easier).

Take off the upper plastic sheet and turn the dough over onto a 10-inch detachable tart pan. Press the dough into the center of the pan, covering the edges and bottom. Take out the leftover plastic and cut off any extra. Freeze for a further ten minutes.

Prepare the unbaked crust according to the recipe's instructions. Alternately, heat the oven to 375°F for a prebaked crust. After lining the tart shell with foil, fill it with pie weights or dry beans.

For ten minutes, bake. Take off the foil and beans, then bake for a further five to six minutes, or until golden. Chill on a rack before to use.

Chocolate Chip-Macadamia Nut Ice Cream Sandwiches Recipe

Net Carbs	Prep Time	Cook Time	Phase	SERVINGS	Protein	Fat	Fiber	Calories
6.8g	300 Min	25 Min	Phase 2	10	11g	47.1g	5g	490.9cal

INGREDIENTS

1/2 cup Butter, salted

3/4 cup Sucralose Based Sweetener (Sugar Substitute)

2 teaspoons Vanilla Extract

3 large Eggs (Whole)

1 cup Atkins Flour Mix (cups)

1/2 teaspoon Baking powder

5 tablespoons Lily's Sugar Free Chocolate Chips

3 cups Heavy Cream

3 large Egg Yolks

1/4 teaspoon Salt

1/2 cup, whole or half Macadamia Nuts

1/2 teaspoon Pure Almond Extract

DIRECTIONS

Turn the oven on to 375°F.

One cup of Atkins Flour Mix is needed for the cookies. Smoothly blend 1/2 cup granulated sugar replacement, 1 tsp vanilla, and melted butter. Once one egg has been added, mix until smooth and thick. Blend in the baking powder and flour mixture until smooth. Add the chocolate chips and fold. Divide the dough into twenty balls of the same size. Place on a pan coated with parchment paper, space them 2 inches apart, flatten a little, and bake for 10 to 12 minutes, or until gently browned. Put aside to cool.

For the ice cream with macadamia nuts: Transfer heavy cream into a 3-quart pot with a heavy bottom and set it over medium heat. To prevent the cream from boiling over, bring to a gentle boil and whisk often. Take off the heat.

Put two eggs, three egg yolks, 1/4 cup sugar substitute, and salt in a big bowl. Beat together with a whisk or a hand mixer until smooth and thickened.

To prevent curdling of the eggs, take about a cup of the hot cream from the pot using a ladle and slowly whisk it into the egg mixture. Whisk the egg mixture and then pour it into the saucepan with the remaining cream.

Place over medium heat and whisk for one to two minutes, or until slightly thickened. Transfer into a sanitized basin, stir in 1 tsp vanilla and almond extract, and let it stand for about 1.5 hours, or until custard has fully cooled to room temperature. Place in the refrigerator for two hours or overnight, covered with plastic wrap.

In the ice cream machine, freeze as directed by the manufacturer. Frozen macadamia nuts should be added 15 minutes before freezing is finished.

To put together sandwiches: Place ten cookies on the work surface, top side down. Working quickly, put 1/4 cup of ice cream on each cookie using an ice cream scoop. Place another biscuit on top of each, bottom side down.

Place plastic wrap tightly over each sandwich and store it in the freezer. For softer ice cream, freeze for at least 4 hours, or overnight for firmer sandwiches. Keeps for up to a month in the freezer.

Atkins Cinnamon Pie Crust Recipe

Net Carbs	Prep Time	Cook Time	Phase	SERVINGS	Protein	Fat	Fiber	Calories
3.1g	10 Min	0 Min	Phase 3	8	7.8g	14.3g	1.9g	172.2cal

INGREDIENTS

1 1/4 servings Atkins Soy-Free Flour Mix
1/4 teaspoon Salt
1 teaspoon Sucralose Based Sweetener (Sugar Substitute)
1 teaspoon Cinnamon
1/2 cup Unsalted Butter Stick
3 tablespoons Tap Water

DIRECTIONS

In a food processor, pulse the baking mix, cinnamon, salt, and sugar substitute until combined. Add the butter and pulse for another 30 seconds or so, or until the mixture resembles coarse meal. Add cold water and pulse until dough barely comes together, approximately 30 seconds. Add an additional tablespoon, if necessary.

Place the dough onto a plastic wrap sheet and shape it into a disk with a diameter of around 6 inches. Tightly wrap in plastic wrap and chill for about half an hour or until solid.

Roll and bake according per pie recipe directions. Yields one pie crust.

Vanilla-Coconut Ice Cream Recipe

Net Carbs	Prep Time	Cook Time	Phase	SERVINGS	Protein	Fat	Fiber	Calories
6.9g	240 Min	5 Min	Phase 2	8	5.3g	43.7g	2g	435.8cal

INGREDIENTS

1 cup Dried Coconut

6 large Egg Yolks

3/4 cup Sucralose Based Sweetener (Sugar Substitute)

2 cups Heavy Cream

1 14 ounces can Coconut Cream

2 teaspoons Coconut Extract

1 teaspoon Vanilla Extract

1/4 teaspoon Salt

DIRECTIONS

For five to seven minutes, toast the coconut in the oven at 350°F, stirring occasionally. Remove from the oven and set aside.

Whisk together the yolks and sugar substitute in a medium-sized bowl.

Heat a medium-sized saucepan over medium-high heat and bring the heavy cream to a simmer. While whisking continuously, slowly add one cup of cream into the yolk mixture. Return the yolk mixture to the pot. We call this procedure tempering.

Cook over medium heat, stirring frequently, for about 3 to 5 minutes, or until mixture is thick enough to coat the back of a spoon. Take off the heat. Add salt, coconut milk, vanilla, and coconut extracts. Relax for four hours.

Fill the ice cream machine with the ice cream mix. Follow the manufacturer's instructions for processing. Add the toasted coconut five minutes before the ice cream is done.

Sweet Potato-Pumpkin Purée Recipe

Net Carbs	Prep Time	Cook Time	Phase	SERVINGS	Protein	Fat	Fiber	Calories
12.2g	20 Min	80 Min	Phase 3	12	2.7g	10.6g	2.5g	159.3cal

INGREDIENTS

3 large Egg Whites

15 ounces Pumpkin (Without Salt, Drained, Cooked, Boiled)

5 tablespoons Sucralose Based Sweetener (Sugar Substitute)

1/2 cup, half Pecan Nuts

1 1/2 pounds Sweet Potato

1/2 cup Heavy Cream

1/2 teaspoon Salt

1/2 teaspoon Pumpkin Pie Spice

1/2 teaspoon Cinnamon

1/4 cup Unsalted Butter Stick

DIRECTIONS

Preheat the oven to 250°F. Grease a baking sheet very lightly.

In a medium-sized mixing bowl, place the egg whites and beat on high speed with an electric mixer until frothy. Add three tablespoons of sugar, substitute gradually, and mix just long enough to produce soft peaks. Transfer onto the ready baking sheet and use a spatula to spread it to a thickness of ¼ inch. Bake for thirty-five minutes. Once the oven is off, let the meringue inside for forty-five minutes. Melt meringue and transfer to a bowl. Mix in pecans with a little toss. Put aside.

Put sweet potatoes in a medium saucepan and let to rest until the meringue is done. Bring to a boil after adding water until two inches over the potatoes. After cooking for approximately 20 minutes or until soft, drain. Turn the heat back up to medium-high. Add the pureed pumpkin, butter, cream, salt, cinnamon, sugar substitute, and two teaspoons of pumpkin pie spice. Mix everything together. Once smooth, mash with a potato masher. Takes approximately a minute to fully heat.

Spoon potato mixture onto a platter, then top with meringue.

Keto Mascarpone Parfait Recipe

Net Carbs	Prep Time	Cook Time	Phase	SERVINGS	Protein	Fat	Fiber	Calories
2g	15 Min	0 Min	Phase 1	4	5.2g	46g	0g	446.5cal

INGREDIENTS

1 cup Heavy Cream

8 ounces Mascarpone

1 tablespoon Sucralose Based Sweetener (Sugar Substitute)

DIRECTIONS

Use an electric mixer with a big bowl and whip heavy cream on medium-high speed until soft peaks form.

Lower the speed to medium and beat in the mascarpone and sugar substitute for 15 to 30 seconds, or until the mixture is smooth. Spoon the cream mixture into each of the four parfait glasses.

If desired, garnish with lemon peel and mint sprigs.

Endulge Keto Chocolate Cups Recipe

Net Carbs	Prep Time	Cook Time	Phase	SERVING	Protein	Fat	Fiber	Calories
3g	20 Min	0 Min	Phase 1	1	1.5g	6.8g	6g	75cal

INGREDIENTS

2 tablespoons Lily's Sugar Free Chocolate Chips

DIRECTIONS

Using a paper cupcake liner, line a muffin pan compartment. Put chocolate chunks into a measuring cup made of Pyrex. 30 seconds at 20% power in the microwave. Repeat this procedure, stirring, until the pieces have melted but retained some of their structure. Blend until the mixture has a smooth consistency.

Apply a layer of chocolate inside the cupcake liner using a pastry brush. Chill for 4 to 5 minutes, or until the chocolate solidifies. Continue until you've eaten all of the chocolate. Peel off the lining gently after the chocolate has solidified.

Cups may be prepared ahead of time, wrapped in plastic, and kept for up to five days in a cool location. To serve this dish at a party, be sure to alter the quantities since it only yields one cup. Also take note that one serving will likely fill two or three small muffin pans. Thus, think about creating smaller cups.

Atkins Chocolate Slushies Recipe

Net Carbs	Prep Time	Cook Time	Phase	SERVINGS	Protein	Fat	Fiber	Calories
4g	5 Min	10 Min	Phase 1	4	2.8g	22.4g	1.9g	229.5cal

INGREDIENTS

1 cup Heavy Cream
1/2 cup Tap Water
2 tablespoons Cocoa Powder (Unsweetened)
1/2 cup Sugar Free Chocolate Syrup
1 teaspoon Vanilla Extract

DIRECTIONS

Cream, water, cocoa powder, and 1/2 cup of unsweetened chocolate syrup should all be combined in a medium pot.

Heat to a boil on a medium setting. Lower the heat to low and cook for five minutes, stirring now and again. Take off the heat and mix in the vanilla.

Pour mixture into two pans for ice cubes. For two hours, freeze.

Place the cubes in a food processor before serving. Pulse until mixture is slushy and coarsely chopped.

Decadent Chocolate Ice Cream Recipe

Net Carbs	Prep Time	Cook Time	Phase	SERVINGS	Protein	Fat	Fiber	Calories
6.7g	240 Min	20 Min	Phase 2	8	7.2g	37.7g	2.7g	388.5cal

INGREDIENTS

3 cups Heavy Cream

2 large Egg Yolks

4 large Eggs (Whole)

3/4 cup Cocoa Powder (Unsweetened)

3/4 cup Sucralose Based Sweetener (Sugar Substitute)

1/4 teaspoon Salt

2 teaspoons Vanilla Extract

1/2 teaspoon Pure Almond Extract

DIRECTIONS

Transfer heavy cream into a 3-quart pot with a heavy bottom and set it over medium heat. Keep it simmering; do not boil. Take off the heat and put it aside.

Whisk together the eggs, yolks, cocoa powder, sugar replacement, and salt in a large mixing basin. Using a rubber spatula to scrape down the sides of the bowl, beat on medium speed for 2 to 3 minutes, or until smooth and thickened. Scoop off approximately a cup of the hot cream from the pan with a ladle, then slowly whisk it into the egg mixture to temper the eggs and prevent them from curdling. Pour the tempered egg mixture into the saucepan with the remaining cream while stirring.

Don't let the temperature rise over 170°F. Place over medium heat and whisk until slightly thickened and coats the back of a wooden spoon.

Transfer into a sanitized dish, blend in the extracts, and let it come down to room temperature, which should take around 1.5 hours. Alternatively, you may put the custard in a sanitized bowl submerged in a bigger bowl of cold water to rapidly bring it down to room temperature. To develop extra flavor, cover with plastic wrap and refrigerate for one additional night, or chill for two hours or until well cooled.

In the ice cream machine, freeze as directed by the manufacturer. Once the freezing process is finished, serve the soft serve ice cream right away, or freeze the firm serve ice cream for two to four hours or overnight in an airtight container. (May be kept for up to a month in the freezer.) Yields about 1 quart; 1/2 cup per serving. Phase 1 approval is granted for this dish; however, the serving size should be lowered to 1/4 cup, or 3.6g NC.

Chapter 7: Tips for Dining Out

You don't have to give up eating out sometimes just because you're following a low-carb diet! Although there aren't usually a lot of low-carb alternatives available at restaurants, you can make practically any entrée into a low-carb meal if you know what to order. These seven suggestions will make dining out guilt-free on a low-carb diet just as simple as cooking at home.

Examine the internet menu of the restaurant before you get there. Prior to sitting down, decide what to get so that you may make an educated and healthful option rather than a snap one.

Before heading out to dine, having a little snack might assist you avoid overindulging at the restaurant. Pick something nutritious and satisfying that won't make you feel hungrier, like some turkey or ham roll-ups or vegetables with guacamole.

To start the meal, many establishments provide baskets of tortilla chips or complementary bread. If you find it difficult to resist the break basket's lure, gently inform the waitress that you don't need it and inquire as to if they may remove it sooner than normal. Ask if you may have sliced vegetables in place of the salsa, hummus, or guacamole that comes with the bread or chips.

When an entrée is served with high-carb sides like macaroni salad, fries, or other vegetables, opt for low-carb options like broccoli or asparagus. Restaurants will often be more than delighted to comply with your request.

Choose your salad components carefully; avoid ordering salads that are served in a shell, such as taco salads, and use sparingly on toppings like tortilla strips and croutons. Furthermore, confirm that any meat you get with your salad is grilled rather than breaded. If you are just starting out on a low-carb diet, stay away from fruits like mangos and grapes that have more carbohydrates.

You may save a lot of carbohydrates when you order a sandwich without the bread or bun. Just ask, and sometimes you can turn a sandwich into a salad or lettuce wrap. If not, stick to the sandwich filling and, if you are in the latter stages of Atkins, remove one slice for an open-faced alternative.

while on a diet and dining out? Order a low-carb omelet or scramble instead of waffles, pancakes, French toast, or even oatmeal. Instead of hash browns or breakfast potatoes, ask for a side order of fresh fruit (berries or half a grapefruit are ideal low carb alternatives).

When dining at Italian restaurants, steer clear of the pasta and pizza areas and instead choose one of the protein-based entrées. For a filling yet low-carb dinner, choose for a recipe that uses chicken, fish, or beef rather than pasta.

Chapter 8: Staying Motivated and Tracking Your Progress

Get acquainted with the Atkins diet. Spend some time learning how the Atkins diet works. Your body will begin burning fat during Phase 1 of the Atkins diet, which may help you lose weight more quickly. Go to the grocery shop after reading this list of approved items for Phase 1.

Establish objectives. Put down your precise weight reduction objective and make a sensible, doable schedule for reaching it. You may stay motivated by setting aside some time to imagine yourself in a better state. Imagine what it would be like to reach your target weight.

Monitor your progress. Set aside time each week or twice a month to celebrate your accomplishments. You may weigh yourself, measure yourself, or just snap a picture of yourself in front of a mirror to monitor your progress. It will be simpler to remain motivated once you begin to realize how far you've come.

Sip a lot of water. Your body may sometimes mistake thirst for hunger. To keep hydrated, drink eight 8-ounce glasses of water per day. Club soda, unflavored soy or almond milk, decaffeinated or normal coffee and tea, and so forth are some more beverages that are permitted for Atkins Phase 1.

Avoid going without food. To keep you full in between meals, Atkins offers a ton of delectable snacks and smoothies. Furthermore, the Atkins diet does not need you to give up all of your favorite indulgences. When your sweet craving strikes, go for an Atkins Nutty Fudge Brownie or Chocolate Candies.

Continue to move. A healthy weight reduction may be promoted by increasing your level of exercise. Every evening, spend thirty minutes strolling around your neighborhood, and use the stairs instead of the elevator at work. Swim in the indoor pool or try a dancing fitness class. Keep up a fitness regimen you love after you've found it. And never forget that little adjustments add up.

Honor modest achievements. Reward yourself with a massage, a lengthy bubble bath, or a fantastic haircut whenever you feel like you've made progress. Make sure to include your close friends and family in the celebration of your accomplishments.

Locate your neighborhood. Take part in the Community Discussions to discuss your struggles and successes with weight reduction. Speaking with other like-minded individuals undergoing similar lifestyle adjustments is beneficial.

Conclusion

A must-have manual for anybody wishing to start a weight-loss and improved living journey is The Atkins Diet Book for Beginners 2024. This extensive book offers a thorough explanation of the advantages of the Atkins Diet as well as its many stages. You'll be well on your way to reaching your health objectives if you adhere to the recommendations and meal plans in this book.

We've studied the fundamentals of the Atkins Diet throughout this book, which emphasizes cutting down on carbs while consuming more healthful fats and proteins. The four stages of the diet—the Pre-Maintenance Phase, the Ongoing Weight Loss (OWL) Phase, the Induction Phase, and the Maintenance Phase—have also been covered. These stages are meant to assist you in achieving long-term success and progressively acclimating to the diet.

A fundamental component of the Atkins Diet is its focus on ingesting low-carb, high-nutrient meals. You may easily make the appropriate diet decisions with the help of this book, which offers a detailed list of foods to consume and foods to avoid. Additionally, it's simple to remain on track and enjoy a variety of delectable meals with the 28-day meal plan and over 50 delicious, healthful, and simple-to-follow recipes.

Many individuals have seen considerable weight reduction in a short amount of time, demonstrating the effectiveness of the Atkins Diet. Apart from aiding in weight reduction, the diet may also lower the risk of heart disease, enhance blood sugar regulation, boost energy levels, and lessen cravings for harmful foods.

As you begin your Atkins Diet journey, keep in mind that perseverance and commitment are essential to reaching your objectives. An excellent tool to help you remain on track and make wise eating selections is The Atkins eating Book for Beginners 2024. You can become a healthier and happier version of yourself if you have access to the appropriate skills and resources.

THANK YOU FOR READING MY BOOK, I APPRECIATE YOUR TIME AND EFFORT.

DO NOT FORGET TO DROP YOUR THOUGHTS ON AMAZON.

THANK YOU…

Atkins Diet FAQs

What does the Atkins Diet entail?

Based on a substantial amount of scientific study, the Atkins Diet® is the original and most popular low-carb weight reduction strategy that offers rapid, efficient, fulfilling, and balanced weight loss. The goal of the Atkins Diet is to "flip the body's metabolic switch" so that fat instead of carbohydrates is burned. Gradual introduction of carbohydrates reduces insulin and blood sugar spikes, which lead to cravings and overeating, ultimately resulting in weight gain.

In addition, Atkins is the preferred weight-loss diet for the millions of individuals with varied degrees of "carbohydrate intolerance," who have a decreased capacity to metabolize carbs.

Each of the four stages of the Atkins 20 diet calls for a gradually increasing carbohydrate consumption. With the help of the plan, a person may determine the appropriate carbohydrate balance for their own weight reduction or maintenance. With so many tasty and healthful food alternatives available, Atkins dieters are inspired to alter and maintain their eating habits.

How can those who follow the Atkins diet plan make sure they are eating a nutritious, well-balanced diet?

The Atkins Diet promotes the intake of a healthy mix of nutrient-dense meals, sufficient protein, a broad range of high-fiber vegetables, low-glycemic fruits, and healthy fats. It also contains a wide variety of foods throughout the whole plan. It teaches each person to find their own ideal ratio of carbohydrates to fat.

Beginning on Day 1 of the Atkins Diet, the focus is on consuming enough fat and protein as well as a broad range of nutrient-dense vegetables to boost the body's ability to burn fat and accelerate weight reduction. This daily vegetable consumption recommendation is much greater than the USDA's recommendation.

As the Atkins 20 Diet is followed, low-glycemic fruits, seeds, nuts, legumes, and finally whole grains are progressively reintroduced back in; the quantity depends on the individual's unique carbohydrate tolerance.

How long can I follow the Atkins 20 Phase 1 protocol?

The longer you limit your daily carbohydrate intake to 20 grams or less, the more body fat you will burn. We advise remaining in this phase until you are within 15 pounds of your target weight.

You may safely go on with Phase 1 based on how much weight you need to reduce, provided that the following three requirements are satisfied:

Your blood pressure, blood sugar, lipid profiles, and blood chemistry are all improving or staying steady and within normal ranges. (To have these levels checked, you will need to see your doctor.)
You are in good health, have plenty of energy, regular sleep cycles, and stable emotions.

You're not disinterested. Boredom might impair your efforts and lead to dishonesty.

But it's crucial to comprehend the Atkins Nutritional Approach in its whole. The program's ultimate objective is for you to proceed from Phase 1 to Phase 2, and then Phase 3, and finally Phase 4, or Lifetime Maintenance, which is your new eating pattern that should last a lifetime. You may discover your unique carbohydrate balance that helps you maintain your current weight and avoid gaining it again by using the techniques outlined below. Changing phases can improve your overall well-being, help you maintain a healthy weight, and lower your chance of developing chronic conditions like diabetes, hypertension, and heart disease.

Having said that, you may continue on Induction for up to six months if you need to lose a significant amount of weight. Naturally, your pace of loss will decrease when you transition to Phase 2. However, if your aim is to lose a moderate amount of weight—let's say 20 to 30 pounds—and you shed the first few pounds quickly, you may choose to follow the Atkins 40 plan. This will help you stop yo-yo dieting and create healthy eating habits that will last for the rest of your life.

How can I tell when to go from one Atkins 20 phase to the next?

There are two choices for when to exit Phase 1.

One possibility is to go straight to Phase 2 in a few weeks. You'll reintroduce nuts and seeds and increase your daily carb intake to 25g net carbohydrates. You will reintroduce dairy products like Greek yogurt, fresh cheeses, and milk, and you will raise your daily carbohydrate intake to 30g as you continue to lose weight. Vegetable juice and beans should then be added again.

You may discover what works for you by going through the balancing process. Knowing your individual carb tolerance is the link between a diet for weight reduction and a diet for life. As you expand the variety of meals you eat, this procedure may need some fits and starts, but it's crucial to comprehend your individual metabolism.

Advantages: You can choose from a wider range of foods; you can transition to a sustainable eating pattern more easily; you have more alternatives for overcoming a plateau since you can always cut down on your carb consumption.

Cons: Slightly slower weight reduction; an increased variety of foods may be too appealing or perplexing.

Choosing to stay in Phase 1 for more than two weeks is your second choice. For the next two weeks, keep eating 20 grams of Net Carbs every day. Consider include nuts and seeds in your list of permitted foods. Because of their high fiber content, nuts have a comparatively low Net Carbohydrate value while being abundant in protein and beneficial fats.

For ease of substitution, replace 3 grams of Net Carbs from other foods with 3 grams of nuts or seeds; however, do not allow your consumption of base vegetables to go below 12 grams of Net Carbs. You may still use your five grams for sauces, sweeteners, dressings, and Atkins bars and smoothies.

As soon as you're within 15 pounds of your target weight, proceed on to Phase 2. It's then time to start adding items further up the Carb Ladder as a means of easing into a permanent eating pattern.

Benefits include quicker weight reduction, more structure, and fewer options, which reduces temptation.

Cons: Boredom; there are no ways to break through a plateau without bringing Net Carbs below the suggested threshold, which may be very annoying and discouraging.

What are some of the health advantages of the Atkins Diet, apart from helping people lose weight?

The Atkins Diet lowers insulin resistance, diabetes, and heart disease risk factors, according to independent third-party clinical studies.

Furthermore, the U.S. Department of Agriculture (USDA http://www.ers.usda.gov/data-products/sugar-and-sw...) reports that the typical American eats about 130 pounds of added sweeteners annually. The Atkins Diet promotes stable blood sugar levels, which reduces cravings for carbs and increases energy, among other health advantages, for everyone (including those without diabetes) who follow it. Studies have repeatedly shown that individuals at high risk for Coronary Artery Disease (CAD) who were on a low-carb diet improved their cholesterol profiles, which reduced their chance of getting CAD.

Adopting an Atkins diet has several advantages for the digestive system as well. Because the Atkins Diet substitutes highly processed, low-fiber carbs with salad greens, fresh veggies, low-sugar fruit, nuts, seeds, and whole grains, it is simple to meet fiber needs. Consumption of fiber is increased by replacing processed meals with an abundance of vegetables in the diet. The greatest strategy to reduce colon-related risk factors is to eat a high-fiber diet. Furthermore, a plethora of scientific investigations has verified that individuals adhering to a high-fiber diet exhibit reduced cholesterol levels and a decreased risk of heart disease in comparison to those following a low-fiber diet.

Is the Atkins Diet suitable for vegans or vegetarians?

With the Atkins Diet, people may eat a broad range of foods as long as they limit their intake of sugar and carbs. One may adhere to a vegetarian or vegan diet. In Phase 2 of the Atkins diet, vegetarians may begin at 30 grams of net carbs and can introduce seeds and nuts prior to berries. Protein-rich foods for vegetarians include cheese, eggs, and soy products. High-protein grains like quinoa, seeds, almonds, soy products, rice and soy cheeses, seitan, and legumes may provide vegans with an adequate amount of protein. Vegans may begin Phase 2 of the Atkins 20 diet at 50 grams of net carbohydrates, which allows them to begin consuming legumes, nuts, and seeds.

While it's well known that the Atkins diet restricts carbohydrate consumption, does it let people consume any carbohydrates at all?

Not a no-carb diet, the Atkins Diet is low-carb. People often confuse Atkins 20's Phase 1 with the whole Atkins regimen. Dieters following the Phase 1 plan are permitted to consume up to 20 grams of net carbohydrates (carbs that affect blood sugar levels; computed as total grams of carbohydrates minus fiber) per day, of which 12 to 15 grams are derived from a variety of vibrant, nutrient-dense vegetables. Following Phase 1, the amount of carbohydrates is progressively raised until the target weight and personal carb balance are reached by each person. In later stages, Atkins dieters may even indulge in whole grains and pasta, depending on how much carbohydrate they can tolerate.

Is Atkins' excessive fat really a criticism?

Atkins emphasizes fat, but a balance of generally accepted healthy fats, such the naturally occurring saturated fats in animal protein, the polyunsaturated fats in vegetable oils, and the monounsaturated fats in avocado and olive oil. People on the Atkins diet may easily eliminate almost all saturated fats if they choose to follow the vegetarian version of the regimen.

It's crucial to keep in mind that consuming more fat is necessary if blood glucose levels are low. The body burns body fat and fat from our diets as fuel when it is in a state known as ketosis, or fat-burning. Protein levels stay consistent throughout the diet but fat intake decreases as you increase your carbohydrate intake.

Over eighty independent peer-reviewed studies have repeatedly shown the safety and effectiveness of the diet.

Does rapidly losing weight pose any risks?

You can lose weight quickly for the first time in your life when you begin the Atkins Induction phase. Remain calm. You lose a significant amount of water weight in the first three to four days, which is what makes the first decrease spectacular. This is because consuming fewer grams of carbohydrates causes blood sugar to surge less often, which in turn causes less insulin to be produced. Your body retains water because insulin causes the body to retain salt, as you are well aware. This cycle slows down as your insulin production decreases, and the result is similar to taking a diuretic. But you will also start to drop body fat after around four days. Those who are young and have a large amount of weight to lose are more likely to join the Atkins regimen and lose weight more quickly.

It's problematic to lose weight too quickly if:

1) You may be losing lean muscle mass as a result of your inadequate diet. Make sure you consume enough calories and eat frequent meals if your goal is to shed body fat solely. When it's not mealtime, have a little snack along with your vitamins. Drink 64 ounces or more of water each day as well.

2) You feel unwell, weak, lightheaded, or worn out. If you're losing weight too quickly, particularly at the start of the program, you could be suffering from an intense diuretic impact. You can lose a lot of water as well as certain electrolytes, which include calcium, magnesium, potassium, and sodium, as a result of this.

Muscle cramps and a heaviness in your legs while ascending stairs are symptoms of electrolyte deficiency. To slow down weight loss and replenish lost minerals, you may need to include extra veggies in your meals and take a supplement of minerals.

However, you're probably not losing too much weight if you feel well and aren't starving yourself. If you're just trying to shed a few pounds, you may want to take your time so that you can finish learning healthy eating practices before moving on to the stages that lead to lifetime maintenance. Just go to Phase 2 and add 5 grams more of carbs to your diet every day. Move onto Phase 3 and progressively increase your consumption in 10-gram increments until weight loss slows to approximately a pound or two per month if you are within five to ten pounds of your desired weight. But if you still have a lot of weight to lose and you have plenty of energy, just rejoice that you are losing weight so quickly.

Why am I unable to consume 20 grams of Net Carbs per day, such as from a peanut butter cup or a piece of whole grain bread, if I am according to the Atkins 20 plan?

This strategy won't work for two reasons. First of all, not all carbs are made equally. The goal of the Atkins Nutritional Approach is to stop blood sugar spikes and excessive insulin secretion, which is a hormone that aids in the conversion of carbohydrates into fat in the body. The first kind of carbs you must reintroduce into your diet after moving beyond. Increase your intake of veggies first, followed by seeds, nuts, berries, then, if you're still losing weight, legumes and grains. Enough refined carbohydrates are present in bread produced entirely of whole-wheat flour for many individuals to experience this insulin-raising, fat-storing impact. You might later have an occasional piece of whole grain bread if your weight reduction is going well and you've upped your daily carb consumption. Regarding the 20-gram peanut butter cup, it has a lot of sugar in addition to hydrogenated fat, which clogs arteries, and sugar is the worst kind of carbohydrate.

Second, the Atkins diet teaches you to consume a range of nutrient-dense carbs for the rest of your life rather than focusing on quick weight reduction. You're getting the greatest benefit for your carbohydrate dollar with these meals since they have the highest concentration of beneficial phytochemicals and antioxidant vitamins in relation to the quantity of carbs. Most individuals are able to enjoy whole-grain bread, fruit, and sometimes even a plate of French fries after they've hit their desired weight and determined their own unique carb balance. Regretfully, the traditional peanut butter cup is just not up to par!

You may want to think about doing the Atkins 40 if you discover that you need more variety and you just need to lose 40 pounds. To learn more, go here.

What is Metabolic Syndrome and "Carbohydrate Intolerance"?

For those with carb intolerance, Atkins is a clinically validated weight reduction and health marker improvement program. The Atkins Diet lowers carbohydrates to start weight reduction, and then it tells the follower to gradually raise their consumption of healthful carbohydrates until they reach their ideal carb balance, or the point at which their body can efficiently digest carbohydrates and sustain their weight over time. No other diet program achieves this.

The initial indication of carb intolerance may be easily identified by measuring your waist, but only a physician can provide a medical diagnosis of this condition. Visceral fat, or fat gathered around the waist, is especially harmful and higher levels of it may be a sign of carb intolerance. Men and women who measure more than forty inches around the waist and more than thirty-five inches around the waist, respectively, may want to discuss carb intolerance with their physicians. Remember that this is only a basic recommendation and that different body types and heights have different health risks.

In Phase I of Atkins 20, are nuts and seeds acceptable despite their carbohydrate content?

Eating no carbohydrates is not the goal of the Atkins diet. It all comes down to consuming the most nutrient-dense carbohydrates while also limiting your consumption. The amounts of fat, protein, and carbohydrates in various nuts and seeds vary. Eating them during the first two weeks of Induction is not advised. However, if you are losing consistently after that, you may try adding some.For ease of substitution, replace 3 grams of Net Carbs from other foods with 3 grams of nuts or seeds; however, do not allow your consumption of base vegetables to go below 12 grams of Net Carbs. You may still use your five grams for sauces, sweeteners, dressings, and Atkins bars and smoothies.

It is important to note, too, that nuts are infamously difficult to consume in moderation. One follows the other until you could have consumed several ounces. Invest in the one- or two-ounce packages to avoid the temptation to overeat.

I'm accustomed to keeping track of calories. On the Atkins Diet, how many am I allowed?

Rather than measuring calories, the Atkins Nutritional Approach calculates grams of carbs. You are permitted 20 grams of Net Carbs throughout Phase 1. Phase 2 involves adding carbs in 5-gram increments as you go toward Phase 3, and Phase 4—the Lifetime Maintenance phase—requires adding them in 10-gram increments at last. We don't need you to track calories while using the Atkins Nutritional Approach. However, we advise you to aim for a healthy range if you're trying to lose weight. That ranges from around 1500 to 1800 calories for women. That ranges from around 1800 to 2200 calories per day for guys. Make sure to restrict empty calories and adhere to the list of meals that are appropriate for the phase you are in at the moment.

There is a definite metabolic benefit to the restricted carb strategy, as shown by research showing that more calories are expended on a controlled carb program than on a low-fat, high-carb diet. However, realize that this does not give you permission to overindulge.

Learning dietary habits that will help you maintain a healthy weight and way of life is the true aim of the Atkins program. This entails breaking past patterns of eating too much, which exacerbated your initial weight issue.

The scale won't go down after I dropped weight for the first few months. How can I break through this wall?

First, pose the following questions to yourself before assuming there is a problem: Do you feel better now? Do your clothing fit you better now? (Because muscle is denser than fat, you could be shedding inches rather than pounds.) If so, is your pace of loss still slowing down? You may only need to keep going a little while longer while making little adjustments. Among them are:

If you are in phase 2, you may try cutting your daily carbohydrate intake by five or ten grams.
If you are eating more than 4 to 6 ounces each serving, you should increase the fat content and reduce the protein content.
identifying and getting rid of "hidden" carbohydrates in processed goods that could also include sugar.
Raising the intensity of your activities.
consuming eight glasses of water, each, on a daily basis.
reducing your intake of cheese, artificial sugars, and extra protein.

What are the advantages of the Atkins Diet for those with type 2 diabetes?

Yes, since the Atkins diet helps manage blood sugar, a type 2 diabetic can overcome high blood sugar. Vegetables heavy in protein, fat, and low in carbohydrates have the least impact on blood sugar, thus they won't elevate blood sugar levels excessively. If someone is using medication to reduce blood sugar, they must consult with their doctor often to modify the dose. When using Atkins, the requirement for medicine decreases significantly and swiftly.

How can I prevent carb creep and what does it entail?

Some individuals start to lose track of how many grams of net carbs they're consuming as they start adding back carbohydrates as they go from Phase 1 into the ever less restricted stages of the Atkins diet. It is probable that you will put the weight back on after that. This is why it's critical to add just one new meal at a time and raise your daily carb consumption by a maximum of five grams each week.

That way, you'll also know right away whether a new meal is making you want unhealthy amounts of food. Keeping a food journal is another strategy for maintaining control as it allows you to identify problematic meals before they become a trigger for binge eating and cravings. For instance, stop eating nuts and observe whether the hunger goes away if, after eating them, you notice that you get hungry again after a few hours.

What sorts of meals are permitted and not allowed on Lifetime Maintenance after I've achieved my ideal weight?

Note that you can consume some of the tastiest foods on the planet while following the Atkins diet. For further information, see the Acceptable Foods Lists. Your metabolism and degree of exercise will determine your carbohydrate threshold, which will determine your unique maintenance program. Males and younger individuals often have faster metabolisms than elderly individuals and females. You may be able to consume whole grains, fruit, beans and other legumes, and starchy vegetables on a daily basis if you have a high tolerance for carbohydrates and engage in frequent physical activity. However, you may need to restrict some of these items if you have a low-carb threshold and are not a highly active person. In either scenario, the focus of your nutrition program will remain on whole foods; sugar, white flour, hydrogenated fats, and a lot of processed foods will be avoided.

What is the daily maximum amount of carbohydrates that is advised for Lifetime Maintenance?

Discovering your own carbohydrate balance is a crucial idea to grasp if you want to keep your weight stable. The ideal amount is the one that prevents weight gain and suppresses cravings and hunger. Everybody has a different carb balance, and you may need to do some trial and error to figure out yours.

Now that I'm in Phase 2, may I have alcohol?

When alcohol is accessible, the body uses it as fuel. Therefore, your body won't burn fat as it burns alcohol. This only delays weight loss; it doesn't halt it. Once the alcohol is consumed, you instantly return to lipolysis since it is not stored as glycogen. However, bear in mind that drinking alcohol might impede weight reduction and make certain individuals more susceptible to symptoms connected to yeast. Once you are off Induction, you may have an occasional glass of wine as long as you include the carbs in your daily total and it doesn't hinder your weight loss. (Approximately 4.3 grams of carbohydrates are present in a 3 1/2-ounce glass of wine.) Spirits like Scotch, rye, vodka, and gin are OK, but don't combine them with sugar-filled beverages like juice, tonic water, or non-diet soda. Diet soda mixers, diet tonic, and seltzer are allowed. Stop drinking alcohol if you have introduced it to your routine and find that you are no longer losing weight.

I was able to follow the Atkins diet with success, but now that I'm in Phase 3, my hunger has grown. How can I handle it and why is that the case?

When you are not in lipolysis (fat burning), appetite may return. Alternatively, you could have included a snack that is making your blood sugar unstable and making you feel hungry or like you're seeking things again. Check to see if anything you recently added has refined grains or sugars in it. Make sure you are getting enough fat and protein on a daily basis. Eat a little bit more if you're eating extra food that satisfies your hunger. If all else fails, discontinue the most recent additions until you manage your hunger.

What kinds of goods and services does Atkins provide?

Atkins offers a large range of goods, resources, and assistance to dieters. Instructions on how to adhere to the diet are provided in the books New Atkins for a New You and New Atkins Made Easy. The New Atkins for a New You Cookbook: 200 Easy and Delicious Low-Carb Recipes in 30 Minutes or Less was published in 2011.

In addition, Atkins provides a selection of frozen meals, protein bars, and shakes that are suitable for a quick lunch, snack, or indulgence. Atkins dieters may indulge in their sweet appetite while controlling their hunger throughout the day since some of these goods are very sweet yet low in carbohydrates. You may buy them at shop.Atkins.com or at major retail outlets. In addition, Atkins provides more than 1,600 recipes, meal plans, and shopping lists for every stage of the plan in its free online community and resource center, Atkins.com. Atkins.com provides community members with all the tools and assistance they need to finish the diet for free; other diets may cost as much as $30 a month. Dieters may get a free quick-start kit on atkins.com upon registering, which provides them with all the necessary information to get started.

How Do Artificial Sweeteners Prevent Loss of Weight?

Artificial sweeteners may produce hypersensitive reactions in a lot of individuals, which may hinder or even halt weight reduction. Since each person is unique, they can all have distinct sensitivities. If your weight loss seems to be stopping, consider how much artificial sweetener you are using and try cutting down.

Why should I stay away from nitrates and nitrites?

Bacon, sausage, and lunch meat often include nitrates or nitrites, which are signs that the food has been cured. Due to the substances used in the process, they can include hidden carbohydrates. Meats that are clearly labeled "No Nitrates/Nitrites" are what we advise eating. Your weight reduction may be halted if you consume more of these hidden carbohydrates than you should each day.

Which book on the Atkins Diet is the most recent?

For everyday wellness, The Atkins® 100 Eating Solution offers simple, low-carb living. Colette Heimowitz's latest book, which delves into the Atkins 100 diet, makes it simple for anybody to adhere to a daily intake of 100 net carbohydrates, enjoy every meal, and see noticeable benefits. The Atkins 100 Eating Solution covers the Atkins 20 and 40 regimens, including low-carb cooking and dining-out methods, and offers a fascinating, appetizing variety of cuisine with 50 delectable dishes and cutting-edge research. The Atkins 100 Eating Solution may assist you with weight loss, diet-related disease management, or just feeling better about your body.

Eat Healthfully, Not Less: Atkins Colette Heimowitz's Your Guidebook for Living a Low-Carb and Low-Sugar Lifestyle emphasizes eating well, not less, for easy weight control and improved general health. Pick the Atkins program that best suits your needs: Atkins 20®, the traditional Atkins method, Atkins 40®, or Atkins 100TM, which focuses on making little adjustments that have a large impact.

Where can I get information and articles on the Atkins Diet?

Go to our SCIENCE and LIBRARY pages for further information about papers or statistics that support the Atkins Diet. For information that you would want to provide to your doctor, please send them to www.atkins-hcp.com, our Healthcare Professional Portal.

Please wait, Your Review is Very Important…

Dear Reader,

I hope this message finds you well. Thank you for choosing to read the Atkins Diet Book for Beginners 2024. Your feedback is incredibly valuable to me, and I would love to hear your thoughts on the book. Whether you've just started, are halfway through, or have finished reading, your perspective matters.

Your feedback is immensely appreciated and will help me enhance future works.

Thank you for taking the time to share your thoughts on the Atkins Diet Book for Beginners 2024. Your support means the world to me.

Happy reading!

Dr. Valerie Kennedy

www.ingramcontent.com/pod-product-compliance
Lightning Source LLC
Chambersburg PA
CBHW080823280726
48660CB00019B/3598